Dr. Bill Akpinar

NO SWEAT? KNOW SWEAT!

The Definitive Guide to Reclaim Your Health

Dr. Bill's Health and Wellness Series

DEDICATION

To my late, dear brother and cherished friend,
Dr. Sylvester Leaks.
Your spirit will always be alive in our hearts.
Thank you.

Illustrations: Janet Hanchey (www.janethanchey.com)
Design & Layout: Apartment One (apartmentone.net)

Dr. Bill's Health and Wellness Series
Shaolin Yoga: Qigong
Zen and the Way of the Sword
No Sweat? Know Sweat! The Definitive Guide to Reclaim Your Health

All medical and health-related information in this book is based on my observations and experience as a physician, dentist, pain management expert, forensic medical examiner, integrative health care provider, and health care educator.

The "About the Author" section demonstrates the extent of my training, as well as my professional degrees and certifications.

— Dr. Bill Akpinar, M.D., D.D.S., Dr.Ac., Ph.D.

CONTENTS

As man develops spiritually, so does his higher mind. He, thus, feels the expansion of his relationship to all of mankind and begins to love his fellow man more and more. It begins to hurt him to see others suffer, and the hurt becomes intensified when he realizes that he may be a contributory cause of their suffering. When this inner pain reaches a certain degree or level, he begins to take steps to remedy it. This represents the evolution of his consciousness and the realization of his enlightenment.

Sometimes, for whatever reason—fear, denial, or personal worldly gain—a person consciously chooses to block these evolutionary steps which will lead to his enlightenment. When this happens, the inevitable "alarm clock" goes off, signaling the wake-up call. It is called karma—or the reality that we reap what we sow. If a person's karmic bank account of credits outweighs the debits, he or she may be able to remain in good standing. Otherwise, the lessons to be learned can appear to be intolerable.

FOREWORD

Dr. Bill Akpinar is not only a man of vision, but also action. Having spent his life in worldwide journeys for the expansion of his knowledge and wisdom, he has devoted himself to a pilgrimage on the road to enlightenment of healing in its many forms, including the study of allopathic, naturopathic, and Eastern medicine. This is no easy task and it would appear that one would have to rise above human limitations to attain this. Many times, to those who truly know him, he does. He has merged all of the conventional and complementary disciplines into a succinct and effective approach to integrated medicine for the well-being of those who seek his services and those who turn to him for educational purposes.

He is a true warrior in the sense of how he has courageously and gracefully managed himself when confronted by the mainstream medical establishment which, though beginning to recognize many people prefer a more holistic approach to their healthcare management, continues to experience reticence when pioneers such as Dr. Bill appear on the scene—despite remarkable healing successes.

Many have probably heard the age-old concept of "Detox or Die." In this latest book by Dr. Bill, he illuminates the much more viable philosophy of "Detox and Live Life to It's Fullest." He also has taken what is considered to be a basic pleasurable and cleansing experience for many, and revealed the universal benefits of sweat therapy as not only an essential physical, mental, and emotional necessity for health, but also a spiritual experience and transformational tool for life. So many today, look for a solution to their health problems such as weight control, stress and sleep disorders, compromised immune systems, organ and glandular imbalances, chronic pain, and other debilitating and degenerative diseases. It is now recognized by scientists and authorities in the health field that environmental and internal toxins such as heavy metals, chemicals, and xenobiotics are a significant and contributing factor in all these conditions. Dr. Bill outlines a simple and effective detoxification approach to eliminate and remove these toxins from our bodies which, thus, leads to purification and optimal health in all aspects and levels of our lives.

With an amazing depth of compassion and energy, Dr. Bill provides us with one more integral body of knowledge and wisdom in this book, to guide our lives in his continued service and dedication to the health of all humankind through natural healing.

Mark D. Smith, ND, PhD, MD

AUTHOR'S NOTE

Fearless, dedicated men and women replete with conviction and faith, have emerged throughout history as beacons of light and inspiration for the rest of humanity, to guide and educate others in areas where they know they have been ordained with the blessing (and burden) of a purpose and mission. Often, their own enlightenment came through intense personal sacrifice, research, discovery, and daring to disseminate the truth. Many endured tremendous pain and suffering (including to themselves and their families), and were usually ridiculed in their chosen path, until the rest of the world acknowledged their contribution.

Without such individuals in the healing profession who had the courage to question and help reform what was considered the "standard of care" of their day, we would, indeed, continue to live in the "dark ages," deprived of their light, guidance, inspiration, and innovation. Although we have succeeded in taking the first steps of a (many) thousand-mile journey, as often quoted by Chinese sages, there is a long, winding road ahead of us. Change is integral, necessary and, perhaps, the only constant in life. May the universe bless, foster, and continue to inspire such individuals and illuminate their paths. This book is but one small step on this long road and is dedicated to such persons of tremendous courage, faith, and resolve. I hope it serves as a small stepping-stone on your own journey of enlightenment.

Prayer for the Physician
Moses Maimonides, 1135-1204

*Before I begin the Holy Work of Healing the creations of your hands,
I place my eternity before the throne of Your Glory that You grant me
strength of spirit and fortitude to faithfully execute my work.*

*Let not desire for wealth or benefit blind me from seeing truth. Deem me
worthy of seeing in the sufferer who seeks my advice—a person—neither
rich nor poor, friend nor foe, good man or bad, or a man in need; show
me only the man.*

*If Doctors wiser than I seek to help me understand, grant me the desire
to learn from them, for the knowledge of healing is boundless. But when
fools deride me, give me fortitude. Let my love for my profession strengthen
my resolve to withstand the derision even of men of high station.*

*Illuminate the way for me, for any lapse in my knowledge can bring illness
and death upon Your creations. I beseech You, merciful and gracious God,
strengthen me in body and soul, and instill within me a perfect spirit.*

Though there are various translations offered of this prayer, this contemporary one appeals to me most. It embraces the heart and soul of what its author intended to keep at the forefront of the minds of physicians, and others, entrusted with the skills and wherewithal to heal or facilitate that process, as well as the trust and faith of those who seek their healing arts and assistance.

Notice the word arts. Health care is both art and science. A balance between the two can engender great strides in both caring for those who are ill and restoration of their health. Healing is sometimes an exact science; but there are times when a physician must go beyond "science" in order to heal the whole person. Problems arise when the arts aspect is forgotten or abandoned, and only the science—especially for profit—is the motivator.

This book offers you both the arts and science of healing the body, following the first sentence in another translation of this prayer: "Almighty God, Thou has created the human body with infinite wisdom." The human body is, indeed, created with an internal infinite wisdom. Yet, there are those solely guided by profits who strive to convince individuals that this is not the case. One hope I have in providing this information to you, is that if you have forgotten or never knew of this wisdom, by the time you finish reading this book, you will change your mind—you will take back your power to participate in the management, and even restoration, of your health and quality of life. It is your right.

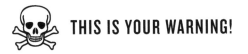

THIS IS YOUR WARNING!

A word of caution:
It may be better that you not read this book if...

• You truly want to believe what health power brokers and media tell you about every area of your life or if you think the importance of detoxification to prevent and heal disease is just nonsense. There are large drug companies, as well as other medical and regulatory organizations, that would be delighted to get you to believe this way. As is said, Just follow the money. If you have already attained enlightenment about these issues, by all means, put this book down now. However, if there is even a remote possibility that your health may not be in balance or you are a person who likes to be proactive about maintaining your health, please keep reading. There is a good reason to believe mankind, in general, will increase its weakened condition in the coming generations because of poor air, water, food, and poisonous emotions. This may become the reality unless... Now is a good time to learn more about how to become deliberate in matters involving your well-being.

• You truly crave the attention and sympathy one gets when ill (especially with a life-threatening disease) and the pain principle serves your pleasure principle in some manner. Chances are, if you do not begin some detoxification program, you will enjoy this dubious privilege. In this case, *"No Sweat? Know Sweat!"* is not for you since once you read it and follow the principles, your body and psyche will get less and less toxic. The result may very well be optimal health. Only you can decide which path you'll travel.

• You don't really care to interact with your grandchildren and, probably, great grandchildren. Who needs them, anyway? They're a drain. Follow the principles in this book, and you'll probably get to know them well and enjoy them more since you'll be healthier and live longer.

• You are an extremely low-tech type of individual who does not wish to partake in the amazing high-technological advances you will see in the next few decades. You'll, most likely, improve your health to the point where you will not only witness, but actually enjoy these advances.

• You don't want to become savvy at investing principle for long-term financial planning, which you will have to master, since you will live a lot longer and have to learn more about trusts, estates, and wills.

Do read this book if you believe...

• My body *is* my business and partner in this life.

• I am a Whole Being and unlike anyone else. Rather than fitting into a statistic, I intend to determine what my unique body-mind-spirit needs in order to be my best.

• I want the opportunity to enjoy life fully, with more vigor and greatly improved health.

This is your "informed-consent" page.

I, the reader of this book, freely and readily consent to read *"No Sweat? Know Sweat!"* and agree to consider the risk(very low)-to-reward(very high) ratio. I am aware that the knowledge provided, possibly against the grain of everything I was taught and was led to believe, may improve and even extend my life. I will be informed of potential complications (very few, but listed in the book's content) and benefits (potential for great health). I realize that by reading this information, I can become the power and force in my life and health; and, that I can begin this process or continue on to a higher level as I take charge of my health.

_____

Signature

Instructions: Sign your name above, then turn the page to start on your path to better health.

"Give me a chance to create sweat, and I will cure disease."
  Hippocrates

NO SWEAT?

This book is going to address the *stinky* topic of sweat. Since you didn't grab your nose and run when you saw the title, you're obviously prepared to hear me out. It's a topic most people don't like to talk about—considered just slightly above events that take place in the bathroom, even though *they* are some of the most important, measurable components involved in your health. Sweat makes an important contribution to human health, as well. It's a sticky subject, to say the least! In fact, sweat, if suppressed and not allowed to take its proper exit, can cause the body to not function at all. The more you suppress it, the more it wants to come out. Yet, in our "proper" Western society, it is not socially acceptable or appropriate (I've always loved that word) to walk around in a state of, let alone speak of sweat. Pharmacies have shelves loaded with deodorants and, worse, "antiperspirants." Society has decided that this natural human process of elimination is to be—well, eliminated. Even at the cost of better health!

If the readers of this book adhere to demographics, the majority are baby-boomers who drank, smoked, and partied hearty through the first half of their lives and finally came to grips, hopefully, with doing what is required to regain and maintain health in the second half. If you managed to toxify the first part of your life or it's been toxified by ways outside your control, which is the inevitable scenario, now you can detoxify the next. Let me begin to explain how.

Certain cultures have dealt, and continue to deal, with body odor (and sweat) in one way or another, whether by moderate means or extremes. Most notable were the French in the last several centuries, who became notoriously famous for immortalizing the highly-coveted "French perfume"—still a hot seller in today's market—in order to suppress and repress the smell of people in crowded Parisian urban settings who had no, or limited, access to baths at that period in time. Steam baths must not have been readily accessible or accessible at all, and their cultural absence is obvious. Today, what is worse is that medical doctors and health clinics conduct a brisk business treating people who "over-sweat"—a condition called *hyperhidrosis*. This one is a doozy, which we'll talk about later in more detail. Browse the Internet or the health section in bookstores, and you'll find a good amount of material on how to medically suppress sweat—akin to holding your breath when near people because you may have mouth odor or deciding to stop eating because you may get gas!

It's noted that Napoleon had a different feeling about body odor. He once wrote a letter to his beloved Josephine in which he advised he would return to her in two weeks and gave her a specific command: "Don't bathe!" Also recorded in history in regard to Queen Elizabeth I, was that she bathed once a month, "...whether she need it or no." There was a period of time when communal baths were all that were available, and bathing was considered a pagan custom that a certain organized religion advised such engagement in could occur once or twice a year, but only if a person absolutely needed it.

We're going to explore the importance of sweat in this book. To do this, we'll take an historical journey into various cultural sweat therapies. As we look at these, we may feel we are more technologically backward than advanced. Once you have all of the information, you can sweat over your own decision as to whether you prefer to hold it in or let it out. You'll learn that when you become tense and nervous in social and other circumstances, your sweat begs to be released through your glands. You'll learn how to detoxify yourself and why even if you attempt to suppress this natural process, which Americans spend hundreds of millions of dollars on annually, it will happen anyway. If you take my advice, you probably won't need to take a change of clothing with you to a more stressful event like a social gathering or business meeting.

The term "No sweat!" is uttered often these days. It implies you sail through an activity with ease, without taxing your nervous system (the sympathetic nervous system, to be precise) to the point of stress and sweat. We also use the phrase, "I didn't even break a sweat." Both might refer to easily maneuvering through some activity, but also may mean that your body is so purified and cleaned out, that not even a life challenge induces you to so much as glisten—much less need a sponge to mop up after you!

Most are aware that humans and animals can smell fear or stress through sweat and act accordingly in anxious or life-threatening situations. This is a kind of fear-factor that seems to leach into our sweat in states of extreme nervousness. You may even have learned to identify a person by the odor of their sweat even if you are not looking at them as they approach. You'll learn in this book, that emotions and conditions of the body influence what sweat smells like, beyond fear or stress, and are often a clue about its state of healthy balance or unhealthy imbalance. **Your ultimate outcome should be odorless sweat.** I'll tell you as much as possible to help you achieve this.

If you deliberately induce sweat on a regular basis, at least two to three times a week, you notice profound changes in the way you feel, as well as how you react to stress. It is your adaptation to stress, or lack thereof, that is a major component to making you sweat against your will. This type of sweat therapy is also referred to as heat or hyperpyrexia therapy, fever therapy, sauna therapy, therapeutic sweating, therapeutic bathing, and possibly dozens of other names.

Let's look at sweat, stress, and movement. It's always a good idea to stretch before we exercise. Why? Stretching pushes the body beyond its normal range of motion and loosens and strengthens muscles at the same time. I'm a bit partial, but the first book in my Dr. Bill's Heath and Wellness Series, *"Shaolin Yoga: Qigong,"* introduces proper breathing techniques, as well as shows how to get maximum benefit from an ancient exercise system with proven, healthful results. Not only are these eight exercises easy to do, but they detoxify the body, mind, and spirit. I highly recommend this book as an addition to sweat therapy and the other protocols suggested in this book.

If you exercise regularly then are subjected to unexpected stress or force, the body can react rapidly and without injury. Regular sweat-therapy induction does the same for the nervous, endocrine, and cardiovascular systems—not to mention the other systems of our bodies. Challenge the body to its healthy limits (or until your face is good and red), and it's a job well done; though as you'll read later, you must learn to pay attention to what your particular healthy limits are in each session—no macho attitude about doing this. The purpose is to heal, not harm your body. Deliberate sweat sessions help you develop a reserve of sorts that is available to you in your normal workday. This reserve lets you keep on keeping on without a need to change garments when faced with a stressful situation. You can literally say, "No sweat!" Sweat therapy is the natural way to deal with what some find to be problematic; and, it's far more holistic than contributing to the profits of doctors or pharmaceutical companies by inhibiting what your body is designed to do to keep you healthy.

You can't put a price on good health, its value is immeasurable. My own experience of working with people, affluent or not, matches the saying that is becoming familiar to many: At the end of one's life, no one says they wished they'd spent more time at the office or worked a bit harder at their job. If you have good health, savor it and do what it takes to maintain it. If your health is not good, do what it takes to restore it as much as possible and maintain that level. Wherever you find yourself health-wise, it requires intention and committed effort on your part. There is no magic bullet for good health; but, of course, as with any health-improving regimen, it is recommended that you check with your physician or health care provider before you embark on this or any other type of therapy. I've watched my patients' lives improve dramatically through sweat therapy, along with other health improvement guidelines.

You'll see some examples in Chapter 12 that demonstrate where the standard medical system fell short and the complementary systems succeeded. Sweat or fever therapy, while it can help cure disease, should not be used instead of medical therapy if some allopathic (standard) treatment is required. That you are reading this book now, shows you have a higher level of sophistication and wisdom about being proactive in regard to maintaining and re-balancing your health and well-being. If your intuition nudges you to consider a form of sweat therapy or other complementary protocols, do your research and make a conscious decision. I can only give you some history, currently-known facts, and personal observations. *Note: Rarely should a person not engage in sweat therapy; and, a few conditions require specific types of sweat therapy. I cover these throughout the book.*

A centuries-old question is, "Is there a doctor in the house?" The answer is a resounding Yes. Your body is your temple, your house. When you decide to become involved in your own maintenance, you've taken a first step to begin a relationship with the world's greatest doctor—yourself. No one knows your body better. No one can feel what you feel or sense what is happening in your body the way you can. If you hope, believe, or anticipate that standard medicine will, indeed, provide your magic bullet for health, you'll miss an incredible opportunity to learn more about what health management means for you—you as an individual—not someone lumped into a statistic.

So many of us are brain-washed by those who seem to be highly-educated people wearing white lab coats. We tend to believe educated means enlightened. We've been indoctrinated to equate lab coats with knowledge, wisdom, experience, and a passion to ease the suffering of individuals. This is not always the case. In medical school, very little time is given to training doctors about lifestyle enhancements and nutrition; and, many believe a simple multi-vitamin is all you need to supplement what they give you. There's no real monetary return for focusing on these basics. And if you speak with some doctors, you learn their reason for getting their degrees and going into practice is rooted in monetary gain and future retirement. (Who wants to re-tire? Aren't you tired enough the first time around?)

When you deal with many mainstream doctors in practice today, you seldom come away with the impression they live to heal and maintain the health of those who entrust their lives to them. Such doctors appear to be a separate species, altogether. But we must be fair and say that some who would like to take a different approach, are under the big guns and watchful eyes of those in the system who do not want them to deviate from the standard practices, ones which the medical establishment refers to as "the standard of care"—the ones insurance will pay for without too much of a fight. The entire allopathic industry is in quite a muddle because there are so many hands grabbing for a piece of the profit pie. And, it's a big, juicy, multibillion-dollar pie at that.

I often wonder what today's standard of care would be had it not been yesterday's mavericks or renegades who challenged, questioned, and dared to think outside the box. Reminds me of Newton's First Law of Motion: "Every object in a state of uniform motion tends to remain in that state of motion unless an external force is applied to it." This principle appears to apply to standard health care.

There is a testament to those who've had the fortitude and guts to say and practice what they believe in their hearts will be good for their fellow man. This testament is an Internet listing called *"Quack Watch."* A health practitioner who has the insight to think outside the box may find him- or herself listed, a dubious honor indeed, on this public (dis)service media tool intended to brand and target practitioners and certain therapies considered "quacks" or quackery. It wasn't that long ago, actually, that chiropractors were considered in this category. Anyone who has ever found a good chiropractor knows how this specialized treatment can restore quality of life and either remove or relieve pain quickly, depending on the medical condition.

The panel members who determine which practitioners should be entered onto this list are doctors and their colleagues. They call attention to agencies to "alert the public" about quack practices. This service is aided by multi-corporate backing. It's understandable that they fear therapies such as energy medicine, the medicine of the future, may actually work and catch on as a legitimate way to view the health paradigm. Behind the profit motive, is a great resolve to discredit practitioners of alternative or integrative methods. One thing these people don't do is seek to learn and understand more about Eastern medicine and philosophies or energy medicine principles. For some, their derisiveness is merely ignorance they have no desire to change. For others, it's a fear of losing control, whether as medical authority figures or profit motivators. Problems occur when alternative therapies prove valid by virtue of individuals healing of even terminal illnesses. Some people who've healed by these means, took them as their sole treatment modality while others used integrative means (allopathic and alternative). But there are those who were told by standard health care practitioners that there was nothing to be done for them; and, this becomes their motivation to explore their alternatives.

There's a phrase used in the world of publicity: It doesn't matter what the media says as long as they spell your name right. Your name being added to this listing is like free advertising for those who dare to be insightful, innovative, and courageous about their health. What's equally intriguing is that members of such panels and other nay-sayers often discretely seek assistance from those they've listed when conventional medicine fails them or their loved ones. I know this from personal experience ("quack-quack!").

I want to offer a disclaimer: Any time you seek the advice or service of a health care practitioner, whether allopathic or alternative, do your research. You do want to be sure you're finding a qualified person to help you manage your health or recovery. Research not only the individual's reputation for quality and success, but the treatment, as well. Integral to successful treatment is trust in the practitioner (preferably one who wants you to be interested and involved) and in the treatment, itself. If you're not comfortable with and confident in either, you won't get the same benefit or result as if you are.

Doctors diagnose illnesses based on symptoms and label them with complex names. It seems the more complex the name, the more credible it is. As with lawyers, what you read appears to be a hieroglyphic, so why try to decipher it? You probably wouldn't understand it anyway. It's designed that way. They give a prognosis and tell you how long you will live unless... God, how I love that one! The "unless" usually involves invasive surgery to remove something your body was designed to need and use, removal of which short-circuits the body's natural bioenergetic pathways, as well as prescribing "proper medications" and their usual, and usually unpleasant, side-effects.

Commercials for drugs are amazing in this regard. They show people, often a couple, enjoying life to the hilt because they take a particular wonder drug. And while the individual or couple or group frolic on your television screen, either a calm, soothing or very, very fast voice talking at warp speed, tells you something like, "Side-effects include nausea, dizziness, gastric bleeding, palpitations, arrhythmia, severe hypertension or stroke, seizure," etc. In other words, you can die while taking this drug! Yes, I want that drug! Now! I want to frolic until I get these complications or die before my time! Makes one feel quite safe.

When you read a drug prospectus, which very few people do, you see warnings for: Cardiovascular thrombotic events; myocardial infarction—which can be fatal; renal papillary necrosis (kidney death)—generally a bad thing; and anaphylactic reaction. The prospectus says that emergency help should be sought for this latter condition. Sure, have an ambulance with paramedics waiting outside your house when you take this. By the way, if true allergic or anaphylactic reactions are not managed within minutes, I guarantee from experience, that there will be death... Your farewell.

I've observed that a great majority of doctors live less than the average person—often with reduced quality of health and life balance. These are the people who tell others how to live when most of their lives are a mess. Some of us doctors, realizing this shortened-life trend early enough in the profession, begin to make lifestyle changes before it's too late. Many I've known, died 10 to 20 years earlier than what is considered the norm for a life span. As an example, both directors of my training program died in their very early sixties, as did several senior attendings. Perhaps this is because they are almost always under the affectations of financial influence by mammoth drug companies, confined by insurance companies, and under constant harassment by lawyers and regulating authorities. These stressors are additional to that of having responsibility for lives. I like to believe they would've traded their expensive send-offs for more years.

Nevertheless, one thing I have always said is, "Doctors eat well!" Every time I visit a doctor friend's office, drug company representatives are swarming all over them like buzzards, collecting and noting data on what type of sushi they should order in for the office next week, or what high-end steakhouse the next "educational meeting" should take place at. Needless to say, "gifts" are becoming so commonplace that new tactics are needed to tie them into education. This has become so rampant, an article appeared in the *New York Times* (Sept. 12, 2006) entitled, "Stanford to Ban Drug Makers' Gifts to Doctors, Even Pens,"—and trust me, the pens are the fanciest looking contraptions I have ever held, and look more like rocket ships than writing tools. The sometimes not-so-hidden message is, "Prescribe these and we will reward you"—a bit like a child getting allowance for doing chores well.

Drug company representatives seem to be hired based on appearance. The men are handsome and the women could be models. I suspect many were former models who also have a brain. And, let's not forget charming... Oh, my God. Many are highly intelligent. I've seen them develop good rapport with doctors, most of whom—chiropractors excluded—are poor business managers. The reps begin to "manage" the doctor's practice, successfully at that. The cornerstone, of course, is promotion of the drug or drugs.

Please understand, I'm not saying not to use doctors (I'm one myself!). Doctors and some allopathic treatments serve a very real purpose. If you break a leg, you don't opt for an herbal concoction as your only treatment. You might use one to help you heal, but you need to get a trained doctor to attend to what a broken leg needs. And, a medicine man holding chicken feathers over your body and chanting, may not be the best treatment for a heart attack. Believe me, I've had enough of these people try to come into my practice as energy medicine consultants. These types are best reserved for photographs you show your friends of your adventurous travels to exotic locales.

There is nothing wrong with your becoming a partner with your physician and learning to trust your inner physician. In fact, both are advisable. You have to use wisdom in your choices; but know there are those who have healed organs affected by disease, even cancer, by detoxifying their body, mind, and/or spirit rather than opting for surgery. I know of a case where an 18-year-old woman was diagnosed with an inoperable brain tumor. Her doctor told her and her parents there was nothing to be done. She walked out of the doctor's office which was located at a major, reputable teaching hospital and went to an M.D. in her town who also used complementary protocols. With Chinese herbal remedies and learning how to push chi (life energy) through her body, she self-healed. No surgery. No drugs. No death sentence. Note: The allopathic system does not like to say a person is cured. If the illness never comes back, they still prefer to use the term *in remission.*

A current example of mainstream medicine's reticence to think "outside the box" is Morgellons Disease where fibers form in skin cells. In summer of 2006, *ABC Prime Time* included a segment on this disease in their national broadcast. People suffering from this debilitating ailment, and dying from it, were labeled by doctors as needing psychotherapy or skin moisturizers. This medical situation broke open when one frustrated mother who was also a research scientist, took a bit of flaky skin from her son's lip and placed it under a microscope and discovered fibers. Further research led her back a couple of hundred years where she found this incident listed in medical journals as Morgellons Disease. Some in the medical community are still arguing against her findings.

What does this have to do with sweat? Sweat therapy is an excellent part of a detoxification program. This may surprise you, but **it can not only play a vital role in disease prevention and treatment, but actually help deter the aging process** (the only real anti-aging agent is death). It is vital that we begin to recognize that much of what we call the effects of aging are actually the impact of toxic accumulations in our bodies over the years. Not to mention what a lack of exercise does to physiology. And, for you doctors who still pooh-pooh this amazing form of health enhancement, here's one from your very own beloved organization: **"Regular use of a sauna may impart a similar stress on the cardiovascular system as running, and its regular use may be as effective (at) burning calories."**—*The Journal of the American Medical Association*—otherwise known as the JAMA (even the lay person has heard of this one). You read this right. This is not the Finnish Medical Association or even the Naturopathic Medical Association. Convincing enough for you?

Ironically, not everyone knows that this organization, the AMA, like its sister-contemporary the American Dental Association, is merely a trade union which began in 1847 in Philadelphia, and NOT a government agency. Just like plumbers' and engineers' unions. And, that's all many of us are—tradesmen working on the human body.

Sweat therapy is one more simple do-it-yourself wellness tool. Join me in the next chapter as we look at what sweat really is.

"Genius is 1% inspiration and 99% perspiration."
Thomas Edison

WHAT IS SWEAT, ANYWAY?

Is sweat so important it warrants a whole book about it? I invite you to read this book in its entirety and make an informed decision.

You may now be asking, "What other secretions, or excretions, will this guy write about next? Urine?" Hmmm...maybe. Surely, sexier secretions could be written about? Of course, some cultures have a different outlook on sweat. There was a time, back in the days of gladiators, when fighters were oiled before they entered the arena. After the "show," the sweat-saturated oil, considered an aphrodisiac, was scraped from their skin and ingested by members of the higher class system and royalty. The belief was that the strength of the fighters, and their virility, were transferred into their sweat and could be absorbed by others. The little blue pill of long ago.

Sweating is as much an essential function for health and well-being as nutrition, breath, and elimination. We get more medical about sweat in the next chapter; but stated simply, sweating regulates our critical body temperature (approximately 98.6°F), keeps skin clean and pliant, and perhaps most importantly, rids our body of wastes. It is estimated that one-third of bodily impurities are eliminated through the skin— our largest body organ. More than one pound of waste product can be eliminated through the skin every day. In fact, *the skin is often referred to as the "third kidney."* Yet, we don't take full advantage of it, as such. Let's explore this so you can better understand why this is.

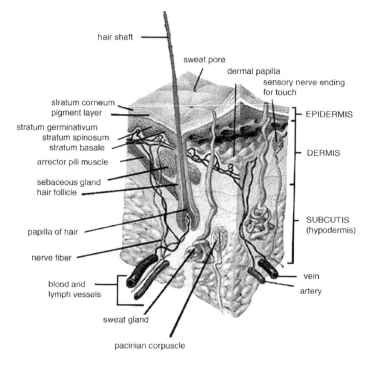

hair shaft

sweat pore

dermal papilla

sensory nerve ending for touch

stratum corneum pigment layer

EPIDERMIS

stratum germinativum stratum spinosum stratum basale

DERMIS

arrector pili muscle

sebaceous gland hair follicle

SUBCUTIS (hypodermis)

papilla of hair

nerve fiber

vein

blood and lymph vessels

artery

sweat gland

pacinian corpuscle

SKIN DIAGRAM

Skin is more complex than the kidneys, or any other organ, with the exception of the brain. It is made up of many elements including nerves, blood vessels, lymph-carrying vessels, hair follicles, sebaceous (oil) glands, pigmentation glands, protective cells, and, of course, sweat glands. Through our sweat glands, the body produces and releases—well, sweat, obviously. Though estimates differ according to differing measuring scales, the body, on average, is 70-percent water. Sweat is 99-percent water. The remaining 1-percent is what gives sweat its unique nature. In this 1-percent, are the toxins and undesirable wastes the body rids itself of as we move through our daily routines. Sweat glands are the kidneys' first cousin in the elimination of substances which do not serve the body. Sweat contains mostly salt (sodium chloride) and urea (a metabolic by-product). This salt is a chemical compound with the formula NaCl, and is found in the extracellular fluid (out of the cells) versus intracellular, which contains a fluid that is mostly potassium.

Salt, essential for life, was used as a form of currency in the Roman Empire. The English word "salary" was derived from the Latin root for salt—*sal salis*. Long ago in Mali, Africa, they put such a premium on salt that this prized substance made a name for itself by immortalizing the expression, "buying its weight in gold;" hence, the legend of the opulent empire of Timbuktu which exported vast quantities of salt. Like anything, too much of a good thing can kill you. Salt is no exception. When we take in too much, we need to get rid of some of it. Sweat is the optimum way to do this.

Someone experiencing adrenal fatigue (hypoadrenia) needs to add salt to their diet. Unless they have high blood pressure, uncommon for those with this condition, salt can actually alleviate symptoms of exhaustion and speed up recovery time. It does this because hypoadrenia usually causes low blood pressure; and in order to raise the energy level, a bit of extra salt is needed. In fact, those suffering from exhaustion that always accompanies this imbalance, are encouraged to add a pinch of salt to their drinking water. There are excellent books available that cover this more fully. But do note that this addition of salt is used in conjunction with a healthy diet recommended for those in recovery. Research is always a good idea.

Urea, the other component of sweat, is an organic compound of carbon, oxygen, nitrogen, and hydrogen. It's formula is CON_2H_4, and is produced from carbon-dioxide and ammonia in the metabolic process called the urea cycle. Elimination of this is necessary because ammonia, as a common waste-product, is toxic and needs to be neutralized. Another end-product is uric acid, which when accumulated in the body, leads to the painful collection of arthritic uric acid crystals commonly referred to as "gout." These are the first signs of this life-disrupting disease. Wouldn't you prefer to sweat these out rather than need to protect your big toe and other joints and be in almost constant, incapacitating pain?

When sweat is dried, it forms crystals. This is a visible manifestation of the crystalline structure of one of the body's fluids due to dissolved salts and other substances. These are considered by some as "liquid crystals." By this, it's suggested that dissolved salts found in body fluids, by virtue of their electromagnetic properties in a crystalline manner, have an ability to maintain and transmit life energy-sustaining charges.

Sweat also contains small quantities of bicarbonate, potassium, and odorants o-cresol (2-methyl phenol) and p-cresol (4-methyl phenol)—which give us the qualities of body odor—as do metabolic by-products of foods, drugs, and beverages. Sweat flushes out heavy metals from the body such as mercury, copper, lead, zinc, and others. Though some of these are integral to health, an overabundance becomes detrimental to wellness. Even a hard-core health fanatic will find a bit extra in his or her body just because they live on Mother Earth at this time. We are constantly exposed to these metals in our environment. Nowhere to run; nowhere to hide.

Also eliminated in sweat is lactic acid—the chemical that is responsible for stiff, achy muscles. In extreme generalized cases of build-up, a condition called fibromyalgia can develop. If lactic acid is not eliminated from the body, we can walk around feeling stiff all day—unfortunately for men, at least, in all the wrong places!

No discussion of sweat would be complete without touching on the favorite topic of most people—sex. Scientists at the University of Pennsylvania and Monell Chemical Senses Center in Philadelphia, found that exposure to male perspiration has a marked psychological and physiological effect on women. Did you hear that one, Dr. Freud? The pheromones in male sweat have shown to have a direct effect on the release of the leutininzing hormone that affects the length and timing of women's menstrual cycles. Wow! (I wonder what this does to the theory that women's cycles align with the woman considered the leader in the group?) There is no doubt that the positive effects of female sweat secretions on the male mind and body will be studied next. Maybe it's not a good idea to give up your weekend social club scene yet. Just wait until you see my up-coming book on Taoist sexology. You'll find a lot of goodies to love there!

Prevent a person from sweating by applying substances which block sweat glands and the garbage collection facility shuts down. It's like your private sanitation department going on strike. We literally drown in our own wastes and can die in a relatively short period of time from waste accumulation. Remember "Goldfinger," the popular James Bond movie? The beautiful maiden (Jill Masterson played by Shirley Eaton) died of "skin suffocation," apparently from being painted head-to-toe in gold—a definite relationship between sweat glands being closed down and death.

Sweat is a factor of heat, of course. Heat, whether in an object or imposed on the body, or by the body, must adhere to the Laws of Thermodynamics. I hated physics until I related it to my understanding of health issues in a practical, tangible way which changed this feeling. For those of you who hated this branch of science as well and broke into a cold sweat just thinking about an exam, or never studied it, there were three laws—until a zeroth law was originated. Simply, heat and work (which includes our desired goal to use energy to create fever and sweat) must conform to the physical principles of changes in temperature, pressure, and volume on physical systems (and biological, such as the body). Thermodynamics is taken from the Greek *thermos*, meaning heat. *Dynamics* means power. Thermodynamics, on a very complex level, describes what goes on in all processes that involve generation of heat (internally) and transference of heat (i.e., sauna). When you begin to "turn on the heat," so-to-speak, you develop the power—as you learn later.

Also, the body—as does the universe—must work in accordance with the Law of Conservation of Energy. The law was considered a primordial seed by ancient Greek philosophers. This was believed by Galileo and many others who followed, and postulates that the total amount of energy expressed as a sum of kinetic and potential energy, is an isolated system and remains constant. Energy can be converted from one form to another, but can never be created or destroyed. If this law were not so, the energy in our bodies would remain constant and we would never be able to derive the benefits of sweat. But, we know that this is not so.

How can we know when our body is out of balance? You can get a clue to this with your own quick, low-tech self-assessment. **If you sweat profusely without effort, sweat in the absence of heat, or experience "ammonia-smelling" sweat, you know that something is wrong and that you are in serious need of detoxification**—even before your $1,000 work-up with your doctor. Don't fault him too much for charging that fee, you know he has payments on his Mercedes to make.

The condition known as *hyperhydrosis* (excess sweating) I mentioned earlier, is a major social problem for many people. Is the body in its infinite wisdom, perhaps, trying to push something out? Treatments for hyperhydrosis range from oral medications called *anticholinergics* that can cause blurred vision; impaired speech, taste, chewing, and swallowing; urinary retention; heart palpitations with maybe even a free trip to the morgue to iontophoresis (using electrical current); botox injections (a form of botulinum toxin which is used to temporarily "paralyze" key parts of associated systems) to—if you're ready for this one—surgery. The latter involves placing a person UNDER ANESTHESIA and a lung is temporarily (hopefully) collapsed. Then, with the aid of a camera, a major nerve—a part of the sympathetic chain, is permanently surgically severed. The goal is to interrupt the signal to the body which causes it to sweat "excessively." This means that you are surgically cutting (ouch) a major nerve plexus in the chest to stop you from sweating—something in the human body's blueprint that serves a specific purpose. Kind of like letting a car battery's cells run dry. Is a free tummy tuck included with this procedure?

As I write this, I'm contemplating a bit of purification for myself in my steam sauna. I'm just a little bit inclined to forego the toxins or the surgeon's scalpel for now. Choices I'm contemplating are, dry sauna or infrared sauna? Eucalyptus or lavender? I want to clear my head before pulling out some medical facts for the more scientific types reading this book. I'm sure they, and you, want a more scientific explanation. So, I'll go activate my brain by improving its circulation and oxygen content with my sweat therapy session and bypass the gingko biloba for now. See you in the next chapter.

"A pint of sweat saves a gallon of blood."
George S. Patton

LET'S GET MEDICAL

Ahhh! The last few drops are off my body. I'm back—feeling better after I released some toxins, increased my brain circulation, and am ready to get into the basics with you. Funny how well this treatment clears one's head! Even if you're not a more scientific type, don't sweat about this chapter (sorry, puns are my weakness). This is really easy stuff and actually interesting, especially if you want to improve your health by gaining a better understanding of it. I promise not to be as stiff with this as my own medical school teachers—many who resembled cadavers for their lack of animation. I will not attempt to cram tons of useless garbage into your mind. Some may consider this a stinky topic, but it will be interesting. That's a promise!

Sweat therapy goes back thousands of years. Then, it was referred to as fever therapy. To better understand the mechanisms of sweating and sweat therapy, let's examine some physiological principles. The temperature of the body's deep tissues, or core, remains essentially constant at 98.6°F under normal conditions, plus or minus 1°F. It is slightly warmer in the day and slightly cooler at night. This conforms nicely to the yin-yang cycle described centuries ago by the Chinese. This changes when we develop a febrile illness or, of course, induce sweat therapy. If we take a nude person and subject him or her to temperatures as low as 55°F or as high as 130°F (in dry air), the core temperature will not vary significantly. At higher temperatures, it will begin to go up slowly. This is where the therapy really begins.

Even cold-blooded reptiles, amphibians, and fish have mechanisms to deal with substances that invade their bodies. When exposed to bacteria-laden water, fish swim upstream to warmer water—which helps to "burn out infection." Lizards bask in the sun in an attempt to "bake" it out of their bodies with the sun's heat—sort of a solar-powered, dry sauna. For mammals, we have a temperature-regulation mechanism that naturally raises our body's temperature, causing us to sweat out any disease-causing substances that have invaded us. Dogs do not have sweat glands, but regulate temperature by panting when overheated to release the extra heat. Maybe this, plus what some dogs eat, is why man's best friend's breath can sometimes melt plastic.

Vigorous exercise or subjection to temperature extremes causes the body to produce heat. Therefore, the body temperature can actually go up to 104°F, or even higher—a condition called *hyperthermia*. When the body temperature falls to 96°F or lower, it's called *hypothermia*. When this happens, the body starts to shiver in order to generate more energy and heat; but if the temperature continues to drop, the shivering eventually stops, along with the functions of the body.

When the rate of heat production in the body is greater than the rate at which heat is lost, the body's temperature rises as a result of this build-up—more heat kept in than let out. Normally, the body's heat production is a result of the metabolism. Inducing the body temperature upward, increases the metabolism. Sweating is the end result of this excess heat production and is regulated by a part of the brain called the *hypothalamus*. Nerves in the front part of this organ (anterior hypothalamus) and the back part (posterior hypothalamus) receive two types of signals: One from the nerves in the periphery that are connected to receptors for warm and cold, and the other from the temperature receptors of blood, actually found in the localized region. Thus, the body has back-up or overlapping fail-safe systems to keep it from over-heating—one nervous-system related, one vascular-system related.

This area of the brain which also controls sleep, mood, blood pressure, oxygen delivery, and toxin removal via the lymphatic system, is responsible for increasing temperature inside the body as it sends out nerve impulses through autonomic pathways (part of the nervous system) to the spinal cord, as well as to the sympathetic nerves (nerves

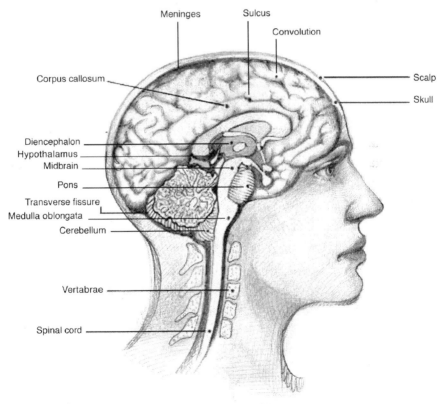

THE HUMAN BRAIN

that connect) found in skin everywhere in the body. This demonstrates why sweating is a function that is facilitated by stimulation of the *sympathetic* nervous system—viewed as the gas pedal normally activated in the "fight-or-flight" response in contrast to the *parasympathetic* nervous system—likened to the brake pedal. Stated simply, when we become nervous, anxious, excited, or agitated, we tend to sweat.

There is a medical legal science which measures degrees of excitation and sweat secretion, along with other parameters, in order to determine if someone who is obviously excited or distressed is telling the truth. This science is often used by non-medical people in order to validate their legal "criminal" hypotheses. As a doctor, I wish lawyers would stick to law and not attempt to be experts in a field for which they have no experience. As a doctor with forensic training and certification, I have seen more than one innocent person unjustly accused as a result of this sometimes flawed measuring system.

It is important to understand even more about the relationship of skin to the body. The skin, along with the subcutaneous (under the skin) tissues, functions as the heat insulator for the body. Fat is the true buffer because it conducts heat only one-third as readily as other tissues. This is one reason why people with a bit extra on them withstand colder temperatures better. I was a skinny runt as a kid who wondered how my older brother, quite plump then, could stay in the cold waters at the beach for extended lengths of time. His skin would remain normal while mine was covered with goose-bumps—like a skinned turkey (I'm from Turkey, so no pun intended!). Skin has almost the same insulating properties as a well-made suit of clothes. The life-threatening down-side of fat storage and toxic substance accumulation, however, is something we'll discuss later.

Under normal conditions, we lose heat from the skin by way of three mechanisms: radiation, conduction, and evaporation. *"Guyton's Physiology"* is recognized as the bible of physiology that medical students must memorize from cover to cover. Mine is so dog-eared and marked up, you can hardly recognize it. According to this reference book, radiation-type heat loss is in the form of infrared heat waves. We lose about 60-percent of our total heat in this way. The wavelengths of these rays are 5-20 micrometers—about 10-30 times the wavelengths of light rays. We are a bunch of radiant creatures radiating heat in all directions. Mosquitoes love this quality about us!

The second form is conduction. About 15-percent of heat loss takes place by conduction to air and about 3-percent to solid objects such as chairs, beds, or other human beings. We are conductors of heat. Just ride a crowded subway at peak times in the summer and you get an up-close and personal experience of this! Along with body heat, you may also get a little eau-de-sweat of garlic, onion, curry, and other residue goodies—especially in a multi-cultural city like New York.

Convection, a form of conduction, represents about 15-percent of heat loss and occurs by convection air currents. Heat is conducted away from the body. If you want to cool off this way, stand naked by the ocean on a windy day. It won't take long at all.

The third form is evaporation. Anyone who sweats on a hot summer day, then cools off, is familiar with this one. It is approximated that a .58 calorie (kilocalorie) of heat is lost for each gram of water that evaporates. Even when we are not sweating, 450-600 milliliters (roughly a quart) evaporates from skin and lungs. When we sweat, this increases dramatically. This is the mechanism we are truly interested in.

When the body is heated, the anterior hypothalamus pre-optic area of the brain is stimulated. Because we do not want to over-heat or need to say, "Stick a fork in me, I'm done," this part of the brain sends a message to the sweat receptors via its autonomic pathways and special nerve fibers called *cholinergic* nerve fibers. These are fibers that secrete a neurotransmitter called *acetylcholine*, and run in the sympathetic nerves (the stimulating ones) along with *adrenergic* fibers. Use this as your next conversation ice-breaker when you meet someone new at a social gathering! They may not break into a sweat over it, but may break into a run—in another direction. Are you still with me? Okay, let's go on.

That was a very technical explanation to simply say that the brain tells the sweat glands to open up so we don't cook to death. Another stress mechanism that will cause a similar occurrence is the release of *adrenaline* and *noradrenaline*—the secretions released as a result of being stressed out.

There are several basic types of sweat glands in the body: The *apocrine* sweat glands located in the armpits and pubis, and to some degree in the nipples and areola—activated by emotional stimuli that releases a scent that can cause sexual arousal (good old Dr. Freud spoke about these on more than one occasion), and the *eccrine* sweat glands. The latter are found mainly in the palms, soles of feet and hairless areas, and in much greater numbers in the body. There are approximately 2-5 million of these in the average person. Although they can be aroused by emotional stimuli (resulting in cold, clammy hands and feet), they are the actual workhorses of the perspiration response. They secrete a clear and normally odorless sweat—in the absence of putrefying bacteria, that is—anywhere from a half-liter to over a liter-and-a-half a day. The milk-producing mammary gland is another type of modified sweat gland. Sweat comes out of the body through all of these glands. Sweat glands are fascinating structures and contain deep sub-dermal coiled portions that secrete the sweat, as well as a duct portion that releases it from the skin. Like many other glands, there is a primary or precursor (initial) secretion released before the sweat. You've probably noticed an initial dampness on the skin before the real sweat starts.

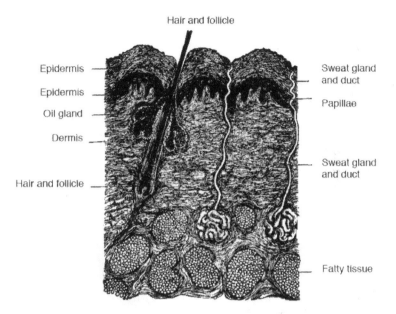

HUMAN SWEAT GLANDS

The odor that originates from the apocrine glands is often a result of putrid skin bacteria such as *corynebacterium tenuis* and *corynebacterium xerosis*. Aromatic compounds in food, spices, and beverages also contribute to this. Most people equate sweat with body odor—sometimes, rightfully so. Interesting research was done on this by Dr. Daniel Paris back in 1974. His paper was entitled, "How much do you stink?" Dr. Paris developed a classification scale of 1 to 10. If you are at the first level, there is minimal odor. At the highest level, people will notice you and probably attempt to move away from you as quickly as possible. Body odor is believed by some researchers, to be related to a *major histocompatibility complex* (MHC) linked to a poorly functioning immune system and is said to be specific to an individual which is why we (and animals) can identify certain people from their odor alone. Among the many factors that influence body odor are diet, medication, occupation, gender, and—drum roll, please—mood.

Although no "scientific data" has been collected on the correlation between the specific odor of sweat and different moods or emotional states such as anger, joy, sadness, excitation, depression, and so forth, I know from personal experience and just being in a small examination room with the many patients who come in with their different conditions, that even if minute, the differences in their particular body odors seem affected by their emotional states. This may also be more evident because people who are in an excited state of mind or on certain prescription drugs or have highly-toxic bodies sweat more which means there's more sweat to smell. (We know animals have the ability to detect fear in humans through this olfactory sense.) The most agitated patients seem to give off the most offensive odors. I can even smell their attempt to mask this odor by hints of deodorants or antiperspirants or colognes that mix with the sweat odor. Anyone in an intimate relationship can usually detect this with a partner, as well. As a personal observation, I've noticed that women generally have a keener sense of smell than men. This is one area where men seem to be "out-gunned."

It's amazing how marvelous the body is. Even as sweat is produced and released to and then from the skin via its tubular canal, the body asks (in about a millisecond), "Do I really want to let all of this out?" By a complex feedback mechanism via messages based on infinite wisdom going back to the brain, the body may choose to absorb some of the substances—mainly sodium and chloride ions—in the event it's been tricked artificially into inducing more sweat than it should, as we would do in sweat therapy. This is how sweat and temperature control are integrally related.

"*Guyton's Physiology*" indicates there are three mechanisms the body uses to reduce heat when the temperature becomes too great:

1. **Vasodilation.** The inhibition of the sympathetic (excitatory) centers in the regions of the brain called the *posterior hypothalamus* (these cause vasoconstriction). The skin's blood vessels become dilated. More dilation means more blood flow. This process transfers heat to the skin as much as eight-fold.

2. **Decrease in heat production.** The mechanisms that cause excess sweat production, such as shivering, are inhibited.

3. **Sweating.** Sweating produces a sharp increase in the rate of evaporative heat loss. When the core temperature goes above 98.6°F, an additional 1-degree-centigrade increase in body temperature causes enough sweating to remove 10 times the basal rate of body heat production. This third one is what we are going to explore thoroughly.

Our bodies have internal heat regulators that go to work for us when we are sick. The result is called fever. Under normal physiologic conditions (non-induced), fever is defined as an increase in body temperature over the normal range and due to a disease process—not from emotion, pregnancy, exercise, environmental exposures, or any other physiologic factors. Fever can be the result of abnormalities in the brain such as a tumor, or of toxic substances that affect the temperature-regulating centers, and can be bacterial or viral in origin.

In Chinese medicine, an integral part of my extended training, the concept of fever or heat is a yang phenomena versus the cool or cold condition called yin. While fever is usually the body's first line of defense during the acute phase of an illness, some insidious microorganisms manage to creep into the body and suppress its fever-inducing mechanism. When this happens, they can lodge into the deeper organs (liver, kidney, spleen, etc.) and slowly wreak havoc in our lives. This is considered a yin illness and can progress from yang to yin as the disease progresses, or begin as a yin disease initially. Western medicine's counterpart to this would be, roughly, acute vs. chronic. This is very dangerous. Syphilis, AIDS, and some types of hepatitis are a few examples. There are times that a febrile type of situation (yang) manages to linger on and progress to the chronic (yin) stage. A steady sweat-therapy and detoxification program can eventually dislodge most of them. Dr. Bill says, "Sweat it out, man!"

The body is structured in such a way that the respiratory system contains hairlike structures called *cilia* that sweep potentially harmful entities, out of the body. The mouth, while rich in bacteria and the most accessible portal of the body, contains a wealth of immune-fighting cells and is considered the body's front-line defense organ. Without this defense mechanism, we could get sick with every kiss (Check out the product I helped develop called Sweet Kiss™ carried by Life Extension Foundation. You'll be amazed at who lives in your mouth! www.lef.org/1.800.544.4440).

One of my favorite scientists was the late Carl Sagan. In his educational series, "*Cosmos,*" he talked about the high probability of intelligent life in other parts of our universe. Perhaps we could consider it a level of human arrogance to believe ourselves the sole inhabitants of an entire universe, as well as that something is not a life-form unless it is identical to ourselves. Sagan's work reminds us that there are 400 billion stars in our Milky Way galaxy with a trillion or so worlds within it. The assumption that life, in any form, did not evolve, even if spontaneously, in a not-too-distant region of space is narrow-minded. We believe time is infinite and that our existence represents not even a millisecond in a hypothetical 24-hour clock of creation and evolution in our universe. If evolution did exist, imagine one or more species that may have begun to emerge and evolve billions of years before us. A parallel may be to consider that most of our highest-tech advancements came about in the last 50 years or so, despite how long we've been around.

When one studies a plausible theory about the beginning of life on Earth as taught to us in college science classes and considers the core elements of phosphorous, sulphur, carbon, oxygen, hydrogen, and nitrogen (I used the mnemonic P.S. Cohn to memorize these), it becomes apparent, to me anyway, there had to be more than just these elements coming together to spontaneously erupt into life in its multitude of forms found on our planet. You may have heard about the likelihood of a tornado blowing through a junkyard and randomly assembling a functional 747 jet. It just doesn't happen. There had to be some organizing force or consciousness involved. This apparent universal organizing force is most often called by various names including the Tao, God, Allah, Elohim, Bhagavan, etc.

I believe, as many other scientists do, that disease-causing entities— viruses, bacteria, parasites—had to resort to a protective slime encapsulation they secrete around themselves in order to be dormant and survive the cold, harsh radiation of space while hitchhiking on meteors, waiting for their next host planet to hatch on and, thus, continue their cycle of perpetuity, as evidenced by their doing so in our bodies.

Which brings us to another sticky topic no one likes to think about: Mucous. Anaerobic organisms hide in mucous slime. This slime is comprised of long fiber-like strands of mucous (thick and ropy) that are calcified or hardened. They can be seen with dark field microscopy whereby a drop of blood is taken from the fingertip and microscopically analyzed. The progressive encapsulation and growth of these strands makes them much thicker than hollow blood vessels. I believe that quite often, these toxin-laden strands, when unable to penetrate blood vessels, clog them and may be the root of many circulatory problems such as heart attack and stroke. These alien-like structures can be found shielding and harboring just about any type of disease-causing entity. Scary looking, indeed!

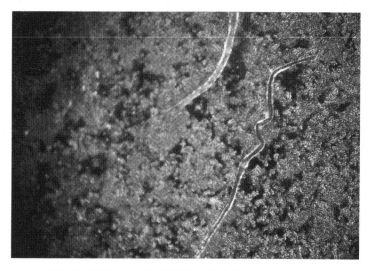

DARK FIELD BLOOD PICTURE WITH CALCIFIED MUCOUS STRANDS

Water is life and we cannot live without it. Any organic entity must have water to survive. It's likely that life forms in other galaxies may need it, as well. Anaerobic organisms have adapted in order to survive the changing phases and challenging environments water is subjected to by virtue of existing in space—an environment constantly in motion either by expansion or spinning, affected by gravity or a seeming absence of it. These organisms exist in the vastness of space, in our biosphere, or in the narrow perspective of our bodies. Their encapsulation in this protective mucous provides them with shelter via frozen water crystals while in space and under certain environmental influences in our bodies.

When one carefully does a dark field microscopic analysis of blood, it is possible to see these strands, some calcified over a span of years. Their length and thickness gives a rough indication of how long they've been around inside the body. For your information, no standard medical tests performed by your physician will show these. Also for your information, this form of analysis is condemned by the mainstream medical community as quackery. (You'll find those who use this analysis on the *"Quack Watch"* listing.) If it walks like a duck, looks like a duck, and quacks like a duck, it's a duck—meaning, the evidence proves the validity of this analysis.

The anaerobic organisms discussed here, have survived for billions of years in the harsh vastness of space where intense radiation, and heat and cold, are the normal environments. Only heat combined with oxygen breaks them apart. When the body is hit with a foreign invader such as a bacterial infection, defender cells called leukocytes, macrophages, and large granular killer-lymphocytes are mobilized and rushed to the scene of invasion. These cells digest the bacterial products and release a substance called *interleukin-1* into the body fluids. This is the body's internal fire-creating mechanism. For you more scientific types, this is also known as *leukocyte pyrogen* or *endogenous pyrogen*.

Notice the word pyrogen—the root pyre means fire—heat. A pyrogen is a substance that causes fever. Exogenous pyrogens come from outside the host, whereas endogenous pyrogens are produced by the host in response to inflammation or infection. The vast majority of exogenous pyrogens are microorganisms and their toxic products which infect the body. These contain a group of molecules which, common to all gram negative bacteria—based on their staining characteristic—is a lipopolysaccharide called *endotoxin*. Gram positive bacteria also create potent pyrogens. Examples are the notorious disease-causing bacteria that belong to the group *streptococcus* and *staphylococcus*, both capable of causing Toxic Shock Syndrome. A minute amount of these are capable of causing fever in humans and, indeed, in a very short period of time.

Generally speaking, exogenous pyrogens act mainly by inducing the formation of endogenous pyrogens through stimulation of two main types of host cells: Those called *monocytes*, a type of white blood cell, and *macrophages*, the body's scavenging cells. Sometimes, there is a fine line between exogenous and endogenous pyrogens, and it's difficult to differentiate which is which.

It has been proven that there is more than one type of endogenous pyrogen. The two classically recognized groups are *IL-1 alpha* and *IL-1 beta*. Since it is now accepted that other cells of the body, aside from the ones mentioned, can produce these as well, a more general term, *cytokine*, has been adopted for these. These cells are also implicated in back pain, as well as joint and muscle pain associated with fevers. This includes the two groups mentioned before, along with *TNF alpha* (tumor necrosis factor), *IFN alpha* (interferon), and *IL-6* (interleukin). Many people have heard of these being used in the field of cancers and viral infections. There is a good reason why. These are all associated with fevers; but, just look at their effect on disease, symbolized by their names, and how creating heat, regardless of the manner, is a protective mechanism for the body. Just as it is an alarm mechanism, it is also a built-in healing mechanism—yin and yang working together, according to Chinese medicine.

When interleukin-1 reaches the hypothalamus, a feedback process is activated that produces fever in as little as a few minutes. It is believed that this is done, initially, by the production of a substance called *prostaglandin*. Prostaglandins can be blocked by preventing the formation of arachidonic acid. This is how substances like aspirin, an antipyretic (fever reducer) work. Since fever has a specific purpose, one should use these fever reducers judiciously and only when truly necessary.

There are many types and variations of "fevers." Dr. Harold J. Jeghers' impressive list includes many; but, here are several I want to give you.

Diurnal Variation: Rhythmic change, with the lowest point in the morning and the highest point in the evening. This seems to make Chinese medicine right when they define yin and yang related, among other things, to time of day and the body's cycles, accordingly.

Psychogenic (Emotional) Fever: An elevation of temperature from stress, but can become chronic if you are always stressed out. The heat produced from living on adrenaline is definitely not good for the body, long-term.

Remittent Fever: Variations not based on dirunal variations, hectic or septic, and intermittent fever—both descriptions for fever periodicity or timing.

Other Fevers: Fever can originate from thirst (thirst fever), malaria (quartan fever where chills and fever occur every third day), biliary (gall) obstruction, Charcot's or hepatic intermittent fever, etc. Fever can be accompanied by chills, ague, or rigor (stiffness). The list goes on and on. Just a note on chills: Chills are a sensation of cold that occur in most fevers. This is created by the central nervous system to call for more heat in order for the body to reach a desired "set point" of temperature—an attempt to return to balance.

We can see that the infinite wisdom of the body creates its own mechanisms to eliminate disease. Perhaps Hippocrates was right. Why, then, don't we choose to create fever and sweat to rid our bodies of disease more often? Why do we and the allopathic health care system try to suppress this natural process? This is within limitation though. Low-grade fever, for a limited period of time, can heal the body. If the body keeps a low-grade fever for an extended time, beyond just a few days or elevates higher and higher, something must be done to reduce it. High fever (over 108°F—though some feel, depending on a person's age, 104-105°F is high enough) has the potential to cook the brain and actually destroy its structure. This results in irreversible neurological damage.

Fever does not come without a cost. For each elevation of body temperature by 1°C, there is a metabolic increase in O_2 consumption by 13-percent, as well as an increase in caloric and fluid requirements. This is significant, clinically, for health care providers monitoring physiologic parameters in the care of ill patients. Patients with very little cardiac or cerebral blood flow may be taxed heavily. This heightened metabolic demand also challenges a developing fetus and is why sweat therapy must be used with extreme caution during pregnancy.

If fever becomes too high, seizures can occur. This is why children with high fever (their thermo-regularity mechanisms are much more sensitive) need to be watched carefully. Anyone with children knows their fever can become dangerously high in the blink of an eye. Sweat therapy, however, does not produce this unless you sit in 150°F+ for an exorbitant amount of time. All you have to do is listen to your body. It will tell you when you're done. Unless you have congenitally-missing sweat glands (very rare), then some form of sweat therapy is for you. Particulars about this are mentioned in the case histories described in Chapter 12.

"The cure for anything is salt water—sweat, tears, or the sea."
Isak Dinesen

A SWEATY PAST:
The History and Mystery of Sweat Therapy

The history of fever induction and, thus, sweat can be traced back to almost the beginning of humanity. Traditionally, sweat rituals were associated with fire. But fire has had to bear the stigma of "burning in hell," causing it to be a subject of fear, power, and mystery. Only sometimes has it been related to "shining in the heavens" or a form of cleansing. Some cultures view it as a symbol of vitality and life. Mikkel Aaland provides a fascinating cultural journey into sweat therapy rituals used around the world in his book, "Sweat." It's a summation of traditions and their foundations for a type of therapy that, as I mentioned earlier, probably existed for as long as we can remember. Aaland, a true adventurer, traveled around the globe for approximately three years in search of the "perfect sweat" protocol. His book even instructs how to build the perfect sauna.

Therapeutic sweating, whether used for medicinal bathing or cleansing rituals, is so ingrained in different cultures, it has been given names. Aztecs named this therapy Nahuatl. The Jews refer to therapeutic bathing as the Switz; the Africans refer to it as the Sifutu; and the Japanese call it the Mushi-buro. Navajo Indians consider the sweat house or lodge, which houses fire, a sacred shrine. Incans believed they were the "sons of the sun." Prometheus believed the

Greeks created civilization by stealing fire from the gods and giving it to humans. The Chinese associate fire with the powerful yang (masculine, expanding) element in their explanation of universal, worldly, and human events in contrast to its opposite, cooling yin (feminine, contracting) counterpart.

Ancient hieroglyphics suggest people wrapped in animal skins, burned fires in caves. Hindus had their own interpretations. Hindu ascetics attempt to gain "inner heat" by meditating near fire. Author and lecturer Joan Borysenko once spoke about monks who dedicate their lives to meditation, striving sometimes for decades to reach the day when they cause their bodies to sweat profusely without any external heat—something, she said, women who experience hot flashes in menopause do naturally (and, I'll add, able to melt an expanse of snow around them on a cold day—the monks, that is—not the women!).

Mankind has consistently tried to attain mastery over fire in order to gain inner strength. Fire walking, a ritual in the South Pacific Islands (and elsewhere these days) is one I participated in several years ago. You place your mind into a highly meditative state, almost trance-like, then walk barefoot for a distance over coals super-heated in the range of 1600-1800°F—and don't get burned. There is no gimmick, no running, no curling the toes. Just slow, steady walking. Talk about the ultimate mind-body connection! And a tribute to our largest organ—the skin.

In the non-high-tech world of yesteryear, fire was the primary method used for sweat and fever therapy. Though not in possession of high-tech tools to measure benefits of sweat therapy on humans, our ancestors instinctively knew its healing properties. They believed spiritual cleansing was a source of healing, that by sweating away "bad spirits," disease could be eliminated. They weren't far off track with this belief.

A somewhat contemporary example of nature innately providing us with a form of sweat therapy is found in Dr. Paavo Airola's book, *"Worldwide Secrets for Staying Young,"* where he tells a story of the Pontine Swamps near Rome, Italy. The swamps were a breeding ground for malaria-carrying mosquitoes. When the Swamps were dried out, the local population managed to eradicate the mosquitoes. While the malaria problem was solved, the next few generations saw an exponential rise in cancerous diseases. Hint: The fever from the malaria killed off cancers! Choose your poison, so-to-speak. Another primitive use of one disease to fight another is the example of treatment of syphilis in early times. Persons who suffered from this ailment were infected with malaria to "burn off" and kill the spirochetes (treponema pallidum) which cause the disease.

Interestingly, there exists today, a tribute to fever in Rome. It is a church, with a tumultuous history, dedicated to "Our Lady of Fever." Not surprising since the Romans had at least three churches constructed as a tribute to her. They were all too familiar with the benefits and destructive capacity of fever through many types of diseases they encountered over time in the lands of their vast empire. I do want to point out that the origins of this Lady and her shrine are a bit more stimulating and came about when the church decided the goddess of erotic sex should undergo a transmutation of sorts. Hardly anyone would argue that sex causes a kind of fever, and if done with "enthusiasm," real sweat.

Benefits of therapeutic sweating seemed to grow parallel to its social importance. Sweat baths in many cultures, were something of a social gathering—a community event where issues of the day were discussed. Sweat baths were associated with purification and rebirth. This is why many cultures included sweat baths as a ceremonial part of marriages, births, and farewells to the deceased and even held the rites at these locations. Sweating is an ancient practice, indeed, for mental, spiritual, and physical cleansing rituals. These older cultures seemed to have believed that the family or community that sweats together, stays together.

Today, when the subject of sauna comes up, many think of Scandinavians. At one time, Scandinavians paralleled the nomadic tribes of Central Asia, moving continuously. As they wandered and eventually settled in Finland, their sweat baths traveled with them. It's a guess, but these sweat baths probably resembled the Native American sweat lodge that could be assembled and dis-assembled as tribes moved from place to place. These earlier sweat therapy users seemed to know what was needed to remain healthy. The Finnish sauna is as much a part of that culture as rye bread is a staple of their diet. Through the history of Reformation, when many bathhouses almost became extinct, the Finnish sauna survived and flourished. Unlike the Swedes and Norwegians who traditionally used saunas for important social events, the Finns saw the sauna not as a luxury, but as a health necessity.

In the Finnish sauna, there is a "kiuas" (stove) which is heated with wood, electricity, oil, or gas. It was originally heated by a smoke sauna, which almost always left behind residual debris from the smoke. The top of the stove is covered by a thick layer of natural stones that radiate heat to the room. Small increments of water are ladled onto the kiuas stones, resulting in vapor rising from the stones called loyly. Bathers use birch twigs (vihta or vasta) to stimulate circulation and alternate cycles of washing and cooling off in the open air. Finns cannot seem to live without a sauna—or, at least, wisely choose not to. According to a research study done in the 1990s, it was estimated there were over 1.5 million of these saunas in a population of 5 million people! In older times, the sauna was known as the "Finnish cure" or "poor man's pharmacy." In fact, Scandinavian doctors are genuinely amazed to see dry, scaly skin conditions of even affluent Western patients when they call on these doctors with a medical problem while visiting these countries. Even the poorest Scandinavians take advantage of the saunas.

Folk-healers practiced their art in this makeshift hospital we call a sauna. Blood drawing, the practice of cupping (to suck the bad blood away) was practiced here, as were magic rituals and births. Long-time president Urho Kaleva Kekkonen was born in a smoke sauna in 1900! For the Finns, the sauna was considered a sacred place. This was not a room for intoxication, bad manners, or sexually indecent behavior. Family members would usually bathe together, whereas, guests would usually bathe with members of the same sex. Since Finland has a cold climate, the hardy ones would cool off by taking a dip in the sea or lake, or roll in the snow. A phrase you may hear often in Finland is, "The sauna is ready."

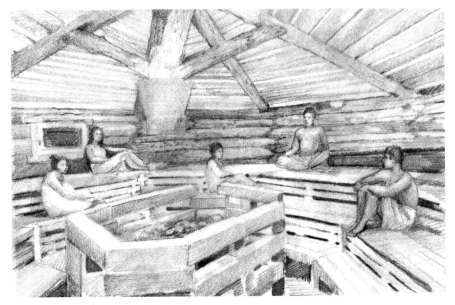

FINNISH SAUNA

Even today in many parts of Finland, it is said that the sauna is designed first, then the house around the sauna. With urbanization, the Finnish sauna (or savusauna) faced major change and near-extinction. Thanks to the Sauna Society of Finland, there are newer, safer versions of the original Finnish sauna all over the world.

Let's look at the Greeks and sweat baths. Being a water-loving culture—handy since Greece is surrounded by water and has approximately 2,000 pieces of prime real estate called "The Greek Islands"—they incorporated the water element into many aspects of life. Water, especially salt water and its related Thalasso therapy, is one of the most therapeutic practices used for centuries.

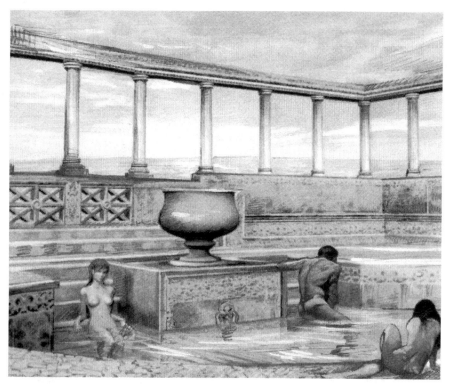

GREEK BATH

It is no surprise that baths and "gymnasiums" flourished during the Greek Empire. Hot tub baths, vapor baths, and hot air baths called laconia, were an integral part of the Greek culture just as ouzo and souvlaki are today. You can imagine the depth of discussions as great philosophers, scientists, and political leaders of ancient Greece gathered in these baths. You can be certain that Plato, Socrates, and other great thinkers used these locations with students and other participants to arrive at, exchange, and discuss concepts still being explored today. And why not, since I will explain how sweat therapy increases brain circulation.

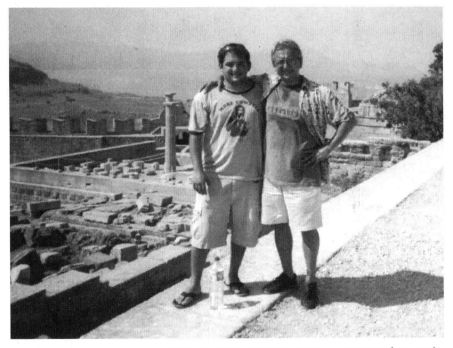

DR. BILL AND SON ADAM AT RUINS OF GREEK TEMPLE WITH BATHHOUSE (RHODES)

Romans, quintessential masters of architectural and other accomplishments on grand scales, used *thermae*—giant baths. Diocletian baths were constructed to handle over 6,000 people at a time and pro-

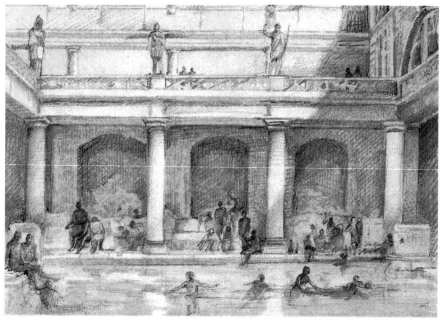

ROMAN BATH

vided the populace with an incredible array of activities from dining to sports to political discussions. Thermae offered every physical, sensual, and intellectual pursuit one could imagine, and there were many. They were cities within cities and accessible to everyone. Emperors were rumored to take baths many times each day. This begs the question: Were their garments simply a matter of style or for convenience of slipping on and off easily?

Aqueducts, a marvelous technological wonder of ancient days, allowed water to be carried over all sorts of terrain to be delivered for use on demand. The Romans were masters of the hypocaust heating system—heating a slab of marble floor and conducting the air via pipes through the walls. Their baths had vaulted ceilings with massive roofs. These exist today in picture-form only. Aside from some vestiges of the original broken-down Greek baths found mostly in the

Greek Islands, and the Roman bath remains found in places like Pompeii, bathhouses of old went into extinction.

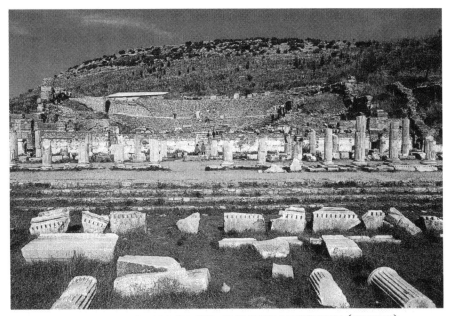

ROMAN RUINS OF ODEUM AND ADJACENT BATHHOUSE (TURKEY)

Perhaps a vestigial remnant of the defunct Roman Empire thrives on the strikingly beautiful island of Ischia, just off of Naples, Italy. There, you find the "Poseidon Gardens" or Giardini Poseidon. I am not trying to make an advertisement for the place, but it is unusual in that there are no less than 22 pools with water temperatures that range from 28°C to 40°C

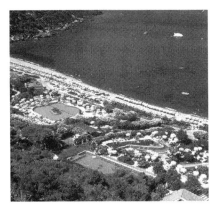

POSEIDON GARDENS

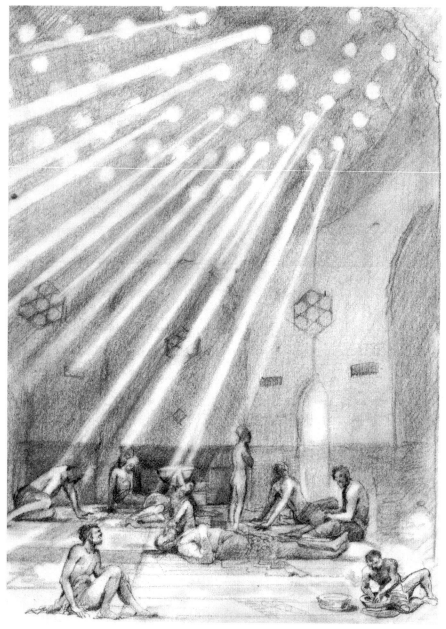

TURKISH BATH (HAMMAM)

(82°F-104°F)—warm, hot, and very hot. These pools share a common characteristic: The water is constantly being renewed thanks to the abundance of natural mineral springs on the island. It is also naturally enriched with "Ischia mud." This is a very fine particulate therapeutic mud with a very high mineral content, that is further filtered for the pool. It is smooth and homogenous, and possesses unique chemical-electrical-therapeutic effects.

The use of such "thermal waters" will greatly enhance health. Not only is the water pure and heated and induces sweating once you get out, it has a high level of sodium, chlorine, potassium, calcium, sulfur, oligo elements, and natural radioactivity. Once you have worked your way up the temperature range, or down if you prefer, you can enjoy a mineralized bath of natural steam comprised of all the elements mentioned here. This takes place in a sauna built into a cave at the very top of the mountain so that you get a great view of the island below. There is also a complete medical facility at the complex that allows you to benefit from all ranges of Western and naturopathic medical treatments, as well. It's a real treat and a wonderful way to detox.

You still have the opportunity to partake in an historical, yet functional Mediterranean sweat bath. To do this, you must travel to the land that shelters the lost ark of Noah and brought the spirit of Santa Claus and the Christmas tradition to the world—Turkey. The Ottoman Empire left a sweaty imprint on the Middle Eastern region. Along with a colorful history, famous scientists, architects, and physicians, you find a means of sweat bathing called the hamam (also spelled hammam) or Turkish bath. Because of its therapeutic properties, the hamam was called the "gizli doctor"—secret doctor—by a famous caliph (ruler). As in other cultures, the wealthy had their own private hamams, whereas the working class used public ones. As mentioned earlier, these were social meeting places for lively debates, gossip, and business transactions.

I have had ample opportunity to sample these. Don't expect the "Arabian Nights" type of images of scantily-clad harem women massaging you and belly-dancing. What you find is a bearded keseci (scrubber), probably named Ahmet or Mustafa, who upon your entry to the bath, takes you firmly by the arm, sits you on the gobek tasi (counterpart of the Roman hypocaust—raised heated marble floor, usually circular), pours water over your head, then starts to scrub you with a rough kese. Your skin is exfoliated in this steamy environment. This is followed by intermittent hot and cool water poured over you in alternating cycles.

Cleanliness is paramount in Islam; so the hamam was favored by religious leaders at the time, especially since it was strongly advocated by Mohammed. Islam also places a premium on modesty. Women's bathing times were different from the men's—no Japanese-like "everyone into the bath" at one time. Trying to buck this trend had the potential danger of loss of body parts, and still is so today! And, rumor was that Jinn, the spirit of caves and dark places, inhabited the hamams. However, it was believed that spiritual thought and behavior would dissipate the Jinn, or evil.

There is an ongoing pilgrimage from rural areas to the city, which means more Turks have access to sauna and steam baths in health clubs, apartment gyms, and individual homes. Modernization is happening more in the Europeanized western part of Turkey, in contrast to Eastern Anatolia which remains more like the "land that time forgot." As this part of Turkey continues to embrace "progress," the popularity of the hamam may go the way of lamb shish kebob at a vegetarian banquet.

No discussion on sweat baths would be complete without mention of our vodka-drinking friends in the former Soviet Union and the Ukraine. They know there is no better way to sweat out the impurities

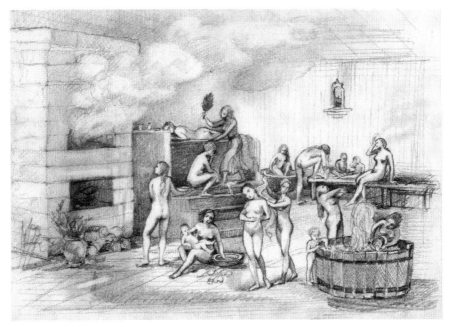

RUSSIAN SAUNA

of the distilled potato liquid than heat. The Russian bania is the steamy counterpart to the sauna and hamam, though bania and sauna development is roughly parallel in northwest Russia, at least. If ever there was a group of people—rich, poor, educated or not—dedicated to the art of sweating, it is the Russians. The cultural link between them and Scandinavians in this area and others, indicates significant parallels regarding what was understood about maintaining health.

Even peasants in the poorest parts of Russia manage to obtain sweat therapy benefits by using clay ovens they crawl into. At the end of the day after bread has been baked, straw matting is placed in the oven on which laborers lie upon and sweat as they crank up the heat and let the heat therapy extract toxins from the body, obviously aware of what most Westerners are ignorant of. From Moscow to Siberia, you rarely meet a Russian who at some time, doesn't take advantage of sweat therapy. It is ingrained in the Russian culture. My visits to the banias were always interesting. These bathhouses, home to the bannik (spirit of the bania), are still quite popular in Russia. The bannik is a fickle mythological creature that inhabits dark, mysterious places. The Russians seem to be particularly careful not to agitate banniks since, like the Jinn, it's believed they could cause quite a lot of suffering for humans.

As Medical Director for the University of Natural Medicine located in Santa Fe, New Mexico, I had the privilege of lecturing to thousands of Russian physicians and scientists, and attended numerous scientific conferences on my various trips to that country. My own roots are in the Ukraine and, thus, being something of a comrade, even if in part, I was welcomed heartily there and recognized for my "courageous exploits" in the field of natural medicine. I love their flair for drama, demonstrated even in their award ceremonies. During one of these trips, the Russian Society of Natural Medicine awarded me with an honorary medical degree. (I can always use some extra blessings. It never hurts.) I say with conviction, that one needs to pre-prime his liver enzymes before such a visit because the legendary Russian affinity for alcohol consumption is accurate. It is considered a personal insult if you do not partake in their several dozen toasts—usually with vodka—made in your honor. Lack of participation results in severe demotion in that culture. Since this was the case that repeated in city after city, I realized at least one rationale for the intense sweat therapy in the land of the czars, one reason they probably consider this the best form of "natural" medicine!

While traditional banias were reformed and modernized (electric heating elements versus wood or coal), the concept is the same: Induce sweat with heat, usually with steam. As with the other cultures mentioned earlier, major life events sometimes take place in these "institutions." After sweating in one of these and de-alcoholing my body—which I needed in a dire way since my level of normal "indulgence" is limited to a glass or two of wine with dinner, I was cheerfully taken out to mounds of fresh snow. Not to be outdone by hearty men aged 70 or older with gold teeth shining at me in anticipation, I took off my shirt and rolled around in the pristine white powder in a temperature 20°F below zero somewhere in a town about 100 miles north of Moscow. When I put my shirt back on, I was handed a small shot of restorative liquid to warm me up—also the locals' favorite stress-reliever. Ah, yes, more vodka. Nastrovia! And the process started its cycle all over again.

Native Americans, and other Indian tribes, practiced (and still do) sweat rituals as part of their spiritual and physical cleansing, deeming such rituals to have marked sacred and religious connective power between peoples and the spirit world. These rituals, sometimes differing widely between various tribes, pervaded cultures from the Alaskan Eskimos, south into the land of the Mayans. As spiritually-based peoples, their goal for ceremonies went beyond cleansing the physical body. Aside from knowing that sweat baths offered a cure for illness and revitalization, spiritual and social connectedness were also provided and reinforced connection to the plant, animal, human, and spiritual kingdoms. The sweat lodge ceremony was so powerful for its participants, the European missionaries, often in their sweat-soaked wool garments, saw this as a threat.

Missionaries and government officials systematically banned the use of the sweat lodge in the late 1880s in Canada and parts of the U.S. Sadly, this broke a chain of continuity that had lasted thousands of years. The profound spiritual and socially-connective aspects of these rituals posed a major threat to the programmed expansionist manifesto of religious conversion of these "red-skinned savages," as they

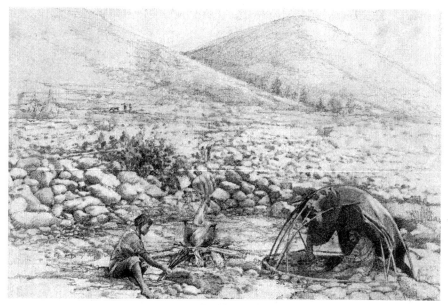

INDIAN SWEAT LODGE

were called, to the "right" path. Luckily, there is a movement to recapture this spirit. In 1995, Irvin Yalom presented his findings on the benefits of interpersonal process-oriented psychotherapy sessions (spiritual therapy, as well) used for troubled teens in a sweat environment at Native American reservations. Thank God for those who strive to keep this great tradition alive!

Immigrants from countries that did not have this practice, must have thought sweat lodges were quite curious, and possibly wondered why anyone would subject themselves to such heat. Many Native American cultures (this includes all of the Americas) used sweat lodges as part of healing ceremonies for those who needed physical, mental, and emotional healing. Certain shamans such as of the Lakota Archie Fire Lame Deer, restrict healing ceremonies to sweat lodges. As odd as it may seem to many Western-trained allopathic health care providers, many Native Americans are willing to stake their health in their time-tested tradition. And, what seems to be of equal importance to them is the peace of mind they derive from their traditions.

Sweat lodge rituals and ceremonies are often done in rounds, with four appearing to be the most common number of these, and are conducted around stones that are heated by fire in front of the entrance to the lodge. Before entering the lodge, there is usually an offering made by sprinkling tobacco onto the fire. The door flap is opened during the prayer sessions to introduce the "grandfathers," or bring the heated stones to the altar—sometimes called the *makakagapi*. This is done by a person specifically chosen for the task, sometimes called a "dog soldier" or "fire man," and is considered a position of honor. Water is poured on the red-hot glowing rocks to pro-

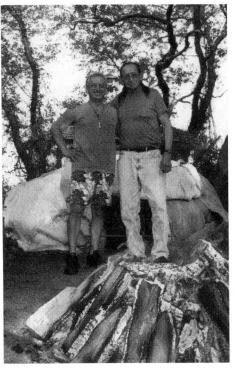

DR BILL WITH MEDICINE MAN BOBBY ONCO PREPARING FOR SWEAT CEREMONY

duce steam that envelops the burning coals, as well as participants. The crunchy vaporized particles can be "tasted" as the steam is inhaled from the red hot stones. In some ceremonies, participants use branches with leaves to lightly beat and stimulate one another. This is akin to any technique used to stimulate the skin and lymph glands prior to doing a sweat therapy. Usually, but not always, men and women partake in separate sweat lodge ceremonies.

There is often chanting, smoking of a pipe (regular tobacco, nothing exotic), praying, drumming, and offerings to the spirit world. The placement (location, according to spiritual principles), orientation (location of the door), construction and materials used, types of offerings, all vary from tribe to tribe. The Sioux consider a sweat lodge's interior representative of Mother Earth's womb; and its darkness, human ignorance. The hot stones coming in are the coming of life; the hissing steam—the creative force of the universe being activated. Many participants ask important spiritual questions and pray for guidance in these revered ceremonies. Quite often, these questions and prayers are answered. One might imagine that when gazing into the hot, glowing red and white stones, images of past relatives or animal spirits appear to offer guidance and encouragement through extraordinary displays of semblances that take form in the steam—like seeing creatures in cloud formations.

I have been given the opportunity to participate in a very sacred healing and sweat ceremony with my spiritual brothers and sisters of the Shinnecock Indian Nation and can say, once again, that the life-transforming aspect of this ritual is unquestionable.

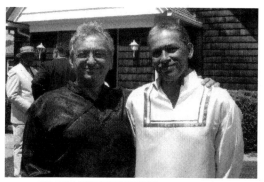

DR BILL WITH REVEREND MIKE SMITH
AT SHINNECOCK INDIAN NATION

Not all minds in the recent past were constricted, since there were a few pioneering souls who, despite the initial ridicule of their peers, knew of the benefits of sweat therapy and used this to help heal patients. If you've ever eaten Kellogg's Corn Flakes® (I loved them as a kid and still do), you may or may not know that Dr. John Harvey Kellogg, for whom the cereal was named, and who probably would marvel at the creative variations of his original formula if he knew just how they'd been changed, was a successful surgeon. At the age of 24 in the late 1800s, he began to run a remarkably successful alternative healing center in Battle Creek, Michigan, and ran it for 67 years until his death at age 91. He was a man ahead of his time with his ideas about health maintenance.

At the core of the program at his health center, visited by people from all over the world, was colonic therapy and, of course, sweat therapy. He called his center the "Sanitarium," which was promoted as "a place where people learn to stay well." He was raised as a Seventh Day Adventist and knew the principles of "healthy living" from an early age. He built on this foundation and, thus, built his extraordinary scientific and humanitarian legacy. No doubt, his several trips abroad where he observed different therapies of the time, helped shape his broader view in the field of detoxification therapy. Had Kellogg emerged today rather in the past, no doubt he'd be included in *"Quack Watch."*

His sanitarium expanded to unheard of proportions. At its peak, it had a staff reported to be between 800 and 1,000, including 30 physicians and 200 nurses and bath attendants who addressed the needs of thousands of patients who passed through or stayed at the dormitory. People waited in line to get the "cure at Battle Creek." It later became a major hospital (Percy Jones General and Convalescent Hospital), then was later used by the U.S. Army as its largest medical installation.

Kellogg's sanitarium was built on sound physiological principles of "biologic living." Dr. Kellogg held more than 30 patents for food products and processes, along with exercise, diagnostic, and therapeutic machines. All along, you probably believed his sole creation was a breakfast cereal! After writing about this, I think I'll indulge in a bowl with some organic soy milk right now to give me some carbs to fuel my brain cells before I continue.

There are intense shamanic ceremonies that endure in South America, primarily in countries that touch the Amazon. I have been fortunate to have participated in such a ritual involving the "vine of the jungle," ayahuasca, also known as the "vine of the gods." The Latin name is *banisteriopsis caapi*. It is an intense experience that usually involves purging (vomiting) and hallucinations, with an end result being amazing insight that is permanent. It is the equivalent of the "Third Eye Opening Ceremony" practiced by shamans in Tibet (my personal experience of this will be presented in an up-coming book). Partaking in these rituals is a prerequisite to become a shaman in South America. Senior shamans explained to me that the arrangement of an individual's DNA informational code becomes favorably influenced by this chemical and becomes naturally reorganized by the plant alkaloids.

Unlike LSD, these are not drugs, but merely indigenous plants that possess the sacred energy of the jungle. While this ceremony normally produces a decent degree of hyperthermia, there is always some level of sweating, depending on the shaman and variety of ayahuasca used. Some of these shamanic or religious ceremonies in other parts of the world involve the use of mushrooms (amanita muscaria). This type of ritual causes transient fever with intense sweating. One has to approach these rituals with extreme caution since they possess a fickle pharmacology and, therefore, the line between a therapeutic dose and a toxic one is very fine, indeed. Severe hypertension and cerebrovascular accident (stroke) can take place—a very bad trip, for sure! Only a trained shaman knows how to carefully choose and process into liquid form, the plants that are appropriate to use in the ceremony vs. those which may be harmful.

The ritual involves a unique pharmacological combination of the ayahuasca, a liana that contains harmaline (an alkaloid) and chacruna (psychotria viridis). These leaves contain the substance known as

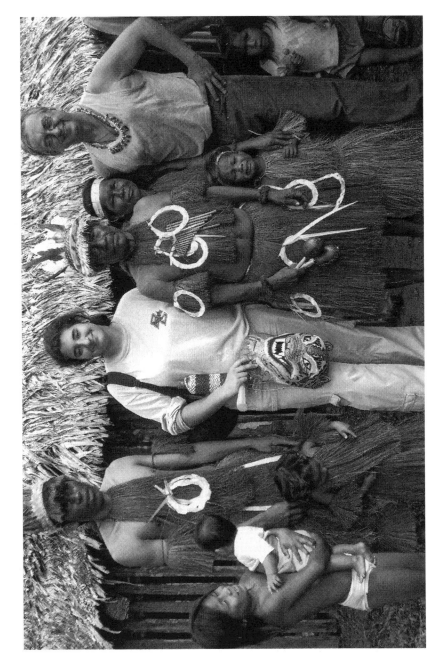

DR. BILL AND DAUGHTER MELISSA WITH SHAMANS IN THE AMAZON.

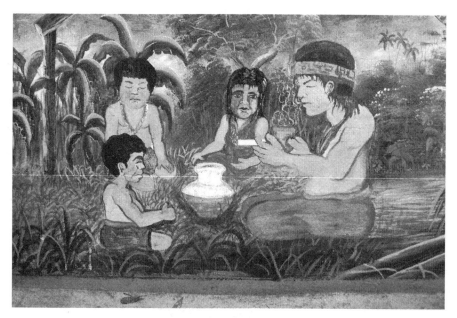

ILLUSTRATION OF AYAHUASCA CEREMONY

DMT. Harmaline is an inhibitor of monoamino oxidase (MAO), a chemical found in synaptic junctions—those connecting spaces between nerves that have been studied extensively by large pharmaceutical companies in the production of drugs for anxiety and depression. MAO normally breaks down the vision-creating compound of DMT before it can cross the blood-brain barrier into the central nervous system. For these combinations to have a vision-inducing and, yes a strongly medicinal property, the mix must be just right—after all, ayahuasca is medicine. It's considered a great medicine by shamans who see disease as primarily a soul-level or energetic manifestation. Shamans believe this medicine frees the soul from its restricted corporeal domain and allows it to temporarily wander the quantum field, to return with, perhaps, a karmic explanation or answer about a disease and even the required treatment.

In China, which I consider my second home, I have experienced yet another sweat therapy technique. Deep in the mountains of Southern China are "spas," although, they would not begin to fit the conventional model of a six-star spa in Sedona, Arizona. After you are greeted, you are taken to a tank filled with heated mineral water from the mountains. It has a brown-tinged color—there is a mix of five to ten different herbs in it—and smells like a Chinese medicine shop one might enter in Chinatown. The herbs used are based on the Five Element Theory of Chinese medicine which has endured for thousands of years. They are blended in a harmonious manner based on wisdom and a safety track record widely studied and categorized. How many other healing systems can make the same claim? Unless abused, I've seen very few complications from using these, and they are quite minor.

After about five minutes in this tank, I realized that the herbs had an exceptional medicinal quality and I began to get somewhat dizzy—many of these herbs can drop blood pressure, as well as blood sugar. I washed off and wrapped up in blankets. A profuse sweat began to take hold and lasted for about 15 minutes. My towels were changed twice. After the treatment, I felt a lightness that was almost euphoric. Remember: Everything diffuses through the skin into your circulatory system. The remnants of the bumble bees, scorpions, and mao tai (the legendary Chinese liquor called "Firewater") left my body with a bang. Given the opportunity to submerge in the ice cold mountain water bath afterwards, I tried it once and only for a short spell. This was enough to bring my heartbeat down to almost non-palpable levels!

India, land of one of my favorite flavors—curry—has yet a different type of hyperthermic or sweat treatment that's been in use for thousands of years. The wealthy elite of pre-Christ India would not even think of considering their mansions complete until their bathhouse, with a fully-functional steam room, was constructed. Indian medicine is believed to have preceded Chinese medicine and has some interest-ing practices, to say the least. One is the *swedana karma*, known as sweat or fomentation practice. Swedana is derived from the Sanskrit word *swid*, which means "to sweat, perspire, and soften." Sweda refers to the internal excreta of the body. Swedana karma, an ayurvedic tech-nique, helps to liquify the sticky doshas that become lodged in periph-eral tissues. Swedanas (herbalized steam baths) are used as part of an ancient ayurvedic purification technique known as *panchakarma*. According to ayurvedic texts, a swedana or steam bath should be given while keeping the head cool and the client in a supine (lying down) position. According to the texts, the shrotas or channels through which biological intelligence flows, must be kept pure and unclogged. A series of deep, internal massage techniques help to assist this. The swedanas soften and melt these toxins so the body can efficiently expel them and are often used with other therapies called *pradhanakarmas*.

Sweating causes fluidity in these doshas so that the sweat glands can sweat toxins out of the system. Two principal means of doing this is with fire and without fire. Fire-induced swedanas include application of hot herbal bolus to a patient, showering the patient with a hot herbal decoction from a pitcher or pot, and a sweat lodge-type cere-mony where special herbs are burned. I have experienced this one in Thailand and found it rather pleasant. Thai culture has the same Buddhistic roots as India and, hence, uses many of the same ayurvedic medicine foundations in its health practices.

There you have it! I've offered here, some of the major sweat cere-monies—some histories and mysteries—offered across time and many lands. For cultural and social traditions to be ingrained in a society, such traditions have to offer a validity that withstands the tests of time. Some genuine benefit must be associated, recognized, and shared for this to happen. Maybe you will use your creativity and come up with your own. You can do a bath using baking soda—a natural detoxifier and skin softener. You can add an essential oil to the water. You can be as creative as you like with your sweat therapies. If life on this planet can sometimes be a sweaty proposition, make it one to your liking and in your favor!

Got any you wish to add to these? Though the actual number of countries in the world is not agreed upon, but generally stated as 193 or 194, I must have left out at least a few techniques!

"To say yes, you have to sweat and roll up your sleeves and plunge both hands into life up to the elbows. It is easy to say no, even if saying no means death." — Jean Anouilh

BENEFITS OF SWEAT THERAPY

Well, we've done some historical and medical reviews of sweating as part of a detoxification protocol. Has reading to this point caused you to work up a sweat yet? If not, perhaps this chapter will get you more in the mood. Let's look at some key benefits of sweat therapy to some major organ systems.

Circulatory, Cardiovascular, and Nervous System Benefits

It is a known fact that people who have cardiovascular fitness live longer. A program of blood pressure reduction and lowering low-density lipoproteins (LDLS) while increasing high-density lipoproteins (HDLS), lowers risk of heart attack and stroke. If we increase our cardiovascular endurance, as well as our respiratory reserve, this can be a life-saver in the event of a highly stressful situation. It's a form of cardiac reserve—like having a bit extra in your checking account in case you need it.

As beneficial as it is to challenge our minds every day, it is equally beneficial to challenge our bodies with exercise so we can look and feel better. Exercise induces a rise in body temperature. Sweat therapy, which has many physiologic parallels to exercise, can help build this reserve and is akin to a cardiovascular workout. During rest, blood-flow to skeletal muscles averages 3 to 4 milliliters-per-minute per 100 grams of muscle. During extreme exercise and sweat therapy, this can rise to between 50 to 80 milliliters-per-minute per 100 grams of muscle. This is a 15- to 25-fold increase. Capillaries which are normally closed or at rest, open up significantly. Pulse is easily increased in a 15- to 20-minute sauna session to between 100 to 150 beats-per-minute. The distance that life-giving, cleansing oxygen and other nutrients must diffuse from the capillaries to muscles and inner organs is lessened. There is a 2- to 3-fold surface area through which oxygen and other nutrients diffuse and metabolic wastes are removed. Toxins are removed from the organs and tissues and are shunted to the largest elimination organ, the skin. If you wish, you can go even deeper into the mechanisms of this process by referring to *"Guyton's Physiology"* and other physiology textbooks.

When we achieve this, the body burns approximately 500 to 600 calories, even up to 800 calories which is the equivalent of running 10 to 15 kilometers—a nicer and more natural addition to a healthy diet program. This means that your Basal Metabolic Rate (BMR) increases. What a great thing. It is estimated that 3,500 calories have to be burned to lose one pound, which means that even if you only burn 500 calories during sweat therapy, you've lost one-seventh of a pound just sitting still. Combine this with exercise... Well, just do the math. Sorry, all you beautiful people with glistening smiles promoting products that are proven to help you lose weight, just read this book!

Remember that cardiac output and arterial pressure also goes up. This is a wonderful increase because the heart's own circulatory system, the coronary arteries, benefit the heart muscle from the increased blood flow and, albeit slight, removal of blood from the organ itself. The normal resting coronary blood flow in humans is about 225 milliliters-per-minute which is 4- to 5-percent of total cardiac output.

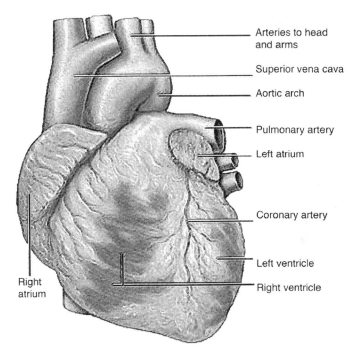

Arteries to head
and arms

Superior vena cava

Aortic arch

Pulmonary artery

Left atrium

Coronary artery

Left ventricle

Right
atrium

Right ventricle

THE HUMAN HEART

When challenged by exercise or sweat therapy, cardiac output can increase 4 to 7 times! You actually feed the heart fresh oxygenated blood through its own two main circulatory components, the left and right coronary arteries. You give them a good workout. Considering that about one-third of all deaths in affluent Western society are due to coronary artery disease—and most of that from ischemic heart disease characterized by diminished blood flow to the heart—it's worthwhile to at least consider sweat therapy. **The 'goo' which narrows the coronary arteries and combines with toxins, heavy metals, and fibrin to form heart attack-causing atherosclerotic plaques, has a greater potential to become liquified and cook out of the body with heat!**

Maybe you're inclined to think, "What the heck, why bother with this? I'll just get a cardiac bypass stent when the time comes." Here's a thought for you. October 21, 2006, was the release date for a broadly-published article called "Doctors Rethink Widespread Use of Heart Stents." I'm sure more research data on this is due to follow. Stents are tiny metal sleeves placed in arteries to keep blood flowing—a quick fix, so-to-speak—and 1.5 million Americans will receive them this year. The article said that "overuse of stents may be leading to thousands of heart attacks and deaths each year." Even the drug-coated ones which are not supposed to clog up, and represent about 85-percent of stents used, lead to *restenosis* which is a tendency for the artery to re-clog. These stents, as well as the surgery, have been responsible for creating repeated problems, including the biggest one—death. **When you make a conscious effort to "take the heat," you may not have to face "taking the knife" later on.**

While we're on the topic of circulation disorders, let's not forget diabetes. This is a disease of faulty sugar metabolism characterized by persistent *hyperglycemia* (high blood sugar levels). There are, essentially, three types: Type I is known as the childhood, or juvenile onset form and is insulin-dependent. Type II is the adult onset form, and unlike Type I, is characterized by insulin dependence and relative insulin deficiency. It is, basically, a disease that results in persistent abuse of the body through poor eating and living habits. The third type, which is often transient, is a gestational form of diabetes. Regardless of the type, chronic diabetes creates damage to blood vessels. When it damages small blood vessels, this is known as *microvascular* disease. Damage to larger vessels, such as arteries, is known as *macrovascular* disease.

According to the Center for Disease Control (CDC), over 60 million Americans are obese. A different agency reports the number of obese and somewhat overweight people in America is closer to 119 million. As obesity rates rise, so does diabetes. The CDC reported a 74-percent rise since 1991. During the same period, diabetes increased by 61-percent. So you see, there is a parallel between poor living and this disease. It doesn't have to be this way.

Chronic blood glucose elevation, as seen in diabetes, creates both types of vessel damage. On the microvascular level, small blood vessels damaged in the eyes leads to marked vision loss, macular edema (fluid build-up), and ultimately, vision loss and even blindness. Microgiopathic retinal organ damage is the most common form of blindness in non-elderly adults in the U.S.

Diabetic neuropathy, or neuropathic disorders (affecting the nervous system), are believed to result from diabetic microvascular injuries to small blood vessels that supply nerves. Nerves deprived of this circulation become, like other organs, injured. In this way, you can see the link between circulatory and nervous system disorders.

Do you enjoy walking or riding a bicycle? Chances are, you may not continue to enjoy these activities for long if you manage to let diabetes get in the way. The prevalence of neuropathy in diabetic patients is estimated to be approximately 20-percent, with neuropathy implicated in up to 75-percent of non-traumatic amputations. I have scrubbed in for many of these types of surgeries, and I assure you, they're not pretty. What is often just a number or a name on a surgeon's printed morning schedule is for the human being getting the amputation, a permanent, incapacitating, and life-changing procedure. His or her life will never be the same again, and may possibly be lived as an invalid.

Diabetic nephropathy is another toll inflicted on the body via this controllable disease. This results when the capillaries of the kidney glomeruli (the capillary tuft), along with a structure called Bowman's capsule that makes up the nephron or main functional filtration unit of the kidneys, become damaged by poor micro-circulation due to angiopathy. The end result, as we examine later, is kidney failure and dialysis.

Thus, the ultimate toll on the body in diabetes is from a damaged circulatory system which affects all systems. This progressive damage can be mitigated, I believe at least to some degree, with a regular program of sweat therapy whether it be through sauna use or some form of sweat-producing form of exercise. And of course, doing both would be better. Don't forget other lifestyle-improving changes while you're at it.

Another significant benefit of sweat therapy is that it helps you look and feel younger. The heat-induced vasodilation, or expansion of blood vessels in the skin's own surface, occurs from the skin's surface expansion as it attempts to accommodate the increased blood flow. This increased blood flow, of course, brings vital nutrients to subcutaneous surface tissue which promotes cellular activity and regeneration. Research has shown that fat located under the skin's sebaceous glands is much more readily emulsified with sweat therapy, thus allowing bacteria and sebum lodged in it to be removed. Regeneration of collagen, the main protein of connective tissue, and loss of which leads to wrinkles and premature aging, is facilitated.

There you have it—your own heat-induced, non-surgical face lift! And by the way, to all of you sun seekers who chased the "perfect tan" on the beaches of Florida, California, or perhaps Hawaii, and now must contend with being a runner-up for a leading role in a remake of Boris Karloff's version of a man wrapped in bandages for thousands of years, you may be able to replace *"The Mummy"* look by hitting the sauna on a frequent basis. Frequent saunas, combined with other lifestyle enhancements, means at least some of that look could probably be replaced by a healthier one.

Fellow men, pay attention to this. Most important to us guys, we can "raise our kundalini" by some significant degree. **There is evidence that far infrared sauna therapy increases nitric oxide levels which can definitely bring some heat to your sex life!** Talk about preserving youth. Viagra, the wonder pill nearly everyone has heard of by now, artificially inhibits the enzyme that normally breaks down nitric oxide, resulting in higher nitric oxide levels. Under normal conditions, the extra nitric oxide helps dilate vital blood vessels. This is significant for its ability to dilate the coronary, carotid, and femoral arteries, which reduces the risk of and helps reverse cardiovascular disease. It will also dilate those vessels so vital for men to keep feeling like men. Studies have shown a 50-percent increase in dilation after only four weeks of far infrared sauna use. Try that one for size! For some extra punch, add L-arginine, the precursor of nitric oxide, to the brew.

Since we're on the subject of sex, a subject I intend to explore like no one's done before in an upcoming book, great sweat-producing sex, especially when expressed through a spiritually-connected relationship, is probably one of the best all-around calorie-burning, invigorating, emotionally-connecting, spiritually-enlightening traditions of all time. It's possible to become the ultimate sexual qigong master (if you follow the right principles, that is) and activate your endocrine, immune, cardiovascular, and every other system you can imagine in a very beneficial manner through sex. Note also that hormone-tinged sex sweat has a uniquely different type of composition from athletic or stress sweat. To experience this, of course, and maintain or reclaim your status as a sexual athlete, it's vital that you "keep up" your sweaty reading by finishing this book. Everything relates to everything else. (My book on Taoist sex will address this and more. Look for it to be in print either this year or the early part of next year, at the latest. I promise it will be unlike any available to date.)

Most of you have seen age spots (lipofuscin deposits which diminish cellular oxygen usage) on people's hands and faces. These also form between the neurons (or nerve cells) in the brain and elsewhere in the body. Beta-amyloid deposition associates with senile plaques in the

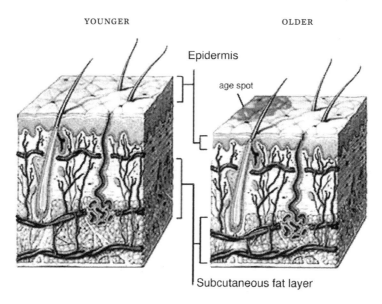

YOUNGER AND OLDER SKIN WITH AGE SPOT

brain, and along with lipofuscin, creates neuronal deterioration. Over time, oxygen utilization and ability to think clearly are affected. Your brain loses approximately .5-percent of white and gray matter a year (authors Copstead and Banasik). This, plus a constantly diminishing blood supply, means the brain loses its means to maintain its own metabolic needs. The function of neurotransmitters is affected.

A neurotransmitter is a biochemical substance, such as acetylcholine or norepinephrine, that transmits or inhibits nerve impulses at a synapse. A synapse is the minute space between a nerve cell and another nerve cell, muscle cell, etc., through which nerve impulses are transmitted from one to the other—like relay stations or posts. Norepinehrine and dopamine (a pleasure-related neurotransmitter) secretion, along with a host of other bio-active substances, are affected. The blood-brain barrier (explained later on) is compromised because the brain doesn't get the "food" it needs. The build-up of metabolic sludge ultimately affects thought processes, memory, and reflexes. Another result is the acceleration of the demise of signals to other organs, therefore, impacting their metabolic functions. In my opinion, you can greatly delay this by detoxifying your brain and nervous system with heat.

Here's something to think about. I've always believed the brain cells can be regenerated and expanded, contrary to the old dogma. This is extremely significant since a concept most people are not aware of is that in the body—which is a biological chain of interrelated, interdependent, and interconnected systems (as is matter in the universe), the chain is only as strong as its weakest link. The quality of function of a particular organ system and, hence, life, can be ruined and perhaps devastated by an imbalance or dysfunction in just one organ system. (The Chinese have this well-documented in their elemental representations of the organs.) For example, a person who develops osteoporosis and takes a bad fall that breaks a hip, is now concerned with the hip and not the relative health of other organ systems. Thus, focus shifts to this system to the detriment of all others. This weakest link now dominates the scene.

Hormones, which are connected to bone health, decline with the results of poor living as we age; and the brain itself (over 90-percent of hormones are regulated by the brain), suffers a decline since it no longer gets needed support as a result of the body's diminished hormone function. All other supportive organ systems suffer a decline, as well—cognitive, metabolic, regulatory. The dog wagging the tail or the tail wagging the dog?

Researcher Arthur Kramer of the University of Illinois, revealed the amazing findings that confirm this in a study reported in the November 16, 2006 *Wall Street Journal*'s *Journal of Gerontology: Medical Sciences.* **Elderly people who take up regular (three hours per week) aerobic exercise (involves increased body heat and sweating) show improved cognitive function after only a few months. Brain volume actually expands!** *This means that the volume of gray matter (the actual neurons) and the white matter (the connectors between the neurons) increases. The age of the mind improves.* The mind is considered part of our conscious and emotional self, but is also part of our physical self in our holistic model. It is very much connected to brain health. An ill mind can create symptoms of anxiety and psychosis.

This neurogenesis has startling implications in cognitive benefits. Learning becomes improved. Multi-tasking, which usually diminishes with age, improves and distractions are weeded out more efficiently. The gray matter found mostly in the frontal lobes (the seat of high-order thinking) gets a good boost, as does the white matter found in the right and left brain's integrating part called the corpus collossum. This expansion assists cognitive efficiency. See the connection? This is believed to take place because of a heightened level of IGF-1 (insulin-like growth factor) that increases blood flow and, more importantly, induces neural stem cells (the progenitor cells) to morph into actual functional brain cells. I always knew it was possible to teach an old dog (or dogma) new tricks!

There almost isn't a person alive who doesn't dread the prospect of age-related mental impairment. Premature aging of the brain is one of the most feared consequences of growing older. It typically begins with short-term memory loss and the inability to learn new information. It eventually progresses to forgetfulness and total impairment marked by senility and dementia. The P300 test measures how fast a

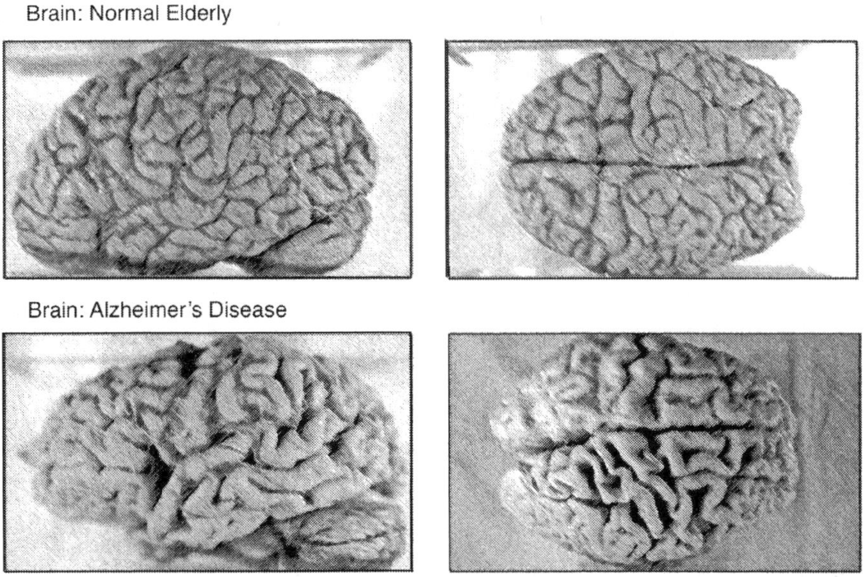

Brain: Normal Elderly

Brain: Alzheimer's Disease

TOP: NORMAL BRAIN SCAN; BOTTOM: BRAIN SCAN WITH NEUROLOGICAL DEGENERATION.

person can generate a single thought (normal time is 300 milliseconds). It slows down about 1 millisecond a year after the age of 20. By the time it reaches 360 milliseconds, senility and dementia are beginning to set in. Dementia, a general term for diseases characterized by nerve cell deterioration, is defined as a loss in at least two areas of complex behavior such as judgment, language, memory, visual or spatial areas, that interferes with a person's daily living. It usually takes a slow, gradual process which unfolds over a period of years. Don't sweat yourself into a panic, however, since many memory changes are temporary and are a result of STRESS rather than physiological change— unless you've managed to infuriate a shaman or insult his family and he puts a curse on you, that is! (A little brevity is a good thing.)

What was I saying? Oh, yeah... The good news is that with the right lifestyle changes, proper nutritional protocols, and increase in oxygen resulting from enhanced cerebral circulation, these can be (whew!) reversed. Open that sauna door, now!

While you're at it, don't forget to consider the brain-protecting, healthy-aging promoters such as *Acetyl-L-Carnitine Arginate* (stimulates growth of brain neurons), *Acetyl-L-Carnitine* (optimizes transport of fatty acids into the mitochondria), *R-Lipoic Acid* along with its counterpart *Alpha Lipoic Acid* that boosts glutathione levels inside the cells and protects from mitochondrial-generated free radicals. *Carnotine* and *Carnosine* are also very potent antiglycation* substances (*destructive cross-linking of proteins and sugar). Of course, as you may know, the B-complex vitamins are the nervous system vitamins, so make sure you add these, as well. These are pointed out, along with other health-enhancing protocols, later on in this book. Adding these is a way you can age well and be well. The Life Extension Foundation is an excellent source of information on this and other related topics.

In addition, mild to moderate *hypertension* (high blood pressure) which affects every organ in the body, benefits from the documented effect of lowering blood pressure through sweat therapy. With sustained hypertension, the risk of cardiovascular disease increases. Arterial walls become thickened and inelastic, unable to expand and contract effortlessly with each heartbeat. Normal blood flow becomes hampered. Life-threatening disease follows. For every incremental increase in blood pressure, your risk of heart attack, stroke, and kidney failure increases greatly.

On the subject of hypertension, the recommended daily consumption of salt as per FDA guidelines (whatever credibility you choose to place into their ever-changing standards—although, here I feel there is some merit) is 2,300 milligrams for young adults and 1,500 milligrams for middle-aged adults, African Americans (who are at higher risk for hypertension), and people with hypertension. For your information, a single serving of a fast-food dinner could, alone, give you more than 2,300 milligrams. Salt, which is used as a preservative, texture provider to food, and as a substance used to mask bland flavor is in everything we consume these days. It seems that there is no way of getting away from it. Despite these recommendations, the average American consumes more than 3,300 milligrams a day, up from 3,100 milligrams a day in 1994, according to the Center for Disease Control and Prevention statistics. An alarmingly great number of people ingest more than 4,000 milligrams per day—routinely. Even the AMA and other groups such as the National Academy of Sciences, Institute of Medicine, and the government's National Heart, Lung, and Blood Institute have cited (for over two decades) the link between salt-induced high blood pressure, which is a significant contributor to heart disease and stroke—the number one and number three causes of death in the U.S. Certain cultures have a predilection for salting foods for various reasons. **Sweat therapy is one of the best ways to rid the body of excess salts that should be removed to maintain optimum health.**

Cancer, by the way, ranks second but appears to be catching up very fast. Some health tips for you to consider here are: Cutting back salt intake (and use either sea salt or the more preferred Himalayan Krystal Salt—a whole different crystal morphology under the microscope), drink plenty of water to dilute ingested salt, and of course KNOW SWEAT! When you indulge in any sweat-producing activity, the salt and toxins are eliminated first. Just taste your sweat for confirmation of how much you may have taken in. Salt will cause water retention and this, in turn, will increase blood pressure and create other problems in the body. People run to doctors to get a "water pill" to push out the excess. Depending on your condition, you may or may not need this. You can certainly help things along by considering your new protocol. As I say, just Know Sweat. I'm giving you a means to help control the number one, number two, and number three causes of death in the U.S. We will touch on cancer in a little while. What have you got to lose, except maybe your excess disease-causing salt, toxins, and perhaps an early meeting with a wills and estate lawyer?

Let me give you more food for thought. Statistics for the U.S. indicate a stroke occurs every 45 seconds and someone dies from stroke every 3 minutes. Worldwide, it's a much higher number. This incapacitating condition known as CVA, or cerebrovascular accident, is the third leading cause of death and disability in the U.S. and Europe. There are, essentially, two types of stroke. The first is ischemic where there is a restriction of blood supply usually caused by a thrombus (blood clot) or embolism, which is the migration of an object from one part of the body to another, creating cerebral blockage. This can be air, fat, bacterial cells, cancer cells, or other toxic debris that haven't been "cooked" out of the body—yet! The second type is called a hemorrhagic stroke. In this type, a blood vessel in the brain that is congenitally faulty or weakened by a disease process, ruptures and leads to bleeding in the brain, itself.

Whatever the mechanism, brain cells deprived of oxygen, die within 60 to 90 seconds. Using a program of heat-induced sweat therapy, along with exercise and better lifestyle management, markedly improves the efficiency of microcirculation, as well as the macrocirculation in the brain and, thus, greatly diminishes the odds of stroke to occur. Heat therapy allows blood vessels to become stronger, more elastic, less brittle, and less susceptible to rupture. Rupture usually is due to an abnormally massive increase in blood pressure such as in a major stress-producing situation...unless your body is conditioned to cope better with such events. Chronic stress and poor lifestyle choices lay down the groundwork for vascular disease that creates this situation.

Therefore, your new "Know Sweat" regimen not only minimizes the risk of sludge and debris being carried and deposited into the brain's circulation system—since much of it will be cooked out on a regular basis with heat therapy—but it will be like a cerebral aerobic exercise, strengthening the arterial system which may have begun to slowly and progressively be compromised by years of deterioration. Not only will the middle muscular layer of the artery, the contractile workhorse called the *tunica media* become healthier by being "tuned up," the outer connective tissue layer, the *tunica adventitia*, and the inner, potentially sludge- and deposit-containing layers (*tunica intima*) will regain or retain health through constant healthy expansion and contraction.

Most people who've had strokes are usually prone to repeat strokes, which can finish things off permanently, especially if health-impairing factors such as poor circulation or hypertension haven't been dealt with properly. A prior history of CVA is not necessarily a contra-indication to sweat therapy if done with caution. You must, of course, check with your doctor or health care provider prior to embarking on this. In fact, such therapy reduces the risk of a repeat incident. If predisposition factors are not dealt with, the chance of a second stroke is quite real. The body is such a magnificent system and will compensate for disease or loss by strengthening the function of the healthier part of an organ (i.e., the opposite side of the brain). **Regaining a healthy, happy, and minimally compromised lifestyle is well within the realm of possibility for anyone who has had a stroke.**

Incidentally, the debate over whether fever therapy procedures can be dangerous to people with blood pressure problems has been ongoing for some time. Many Scandinavian doctors, usually connoisseurs of sweat therapy themselves, express no major concern on this issue. This is probably because heat causes the tiny vessels in skin to expand to accommodate excess blood flow. There is also an increase in nitric oxide, mentioned before, which in itself, dilates blood vessels and lowers blood pressure. An area to exercise a much greater degree of caution is *congestive heart failure.* Heat tolerance is severely diminished in these patients. With this, and some other conditions, very slow detoxifying with low levels of initial heat should be used. An infrared sauna is ideal for this, and best if monitored by a qualified health care practitioner experienced in this matter.

Dr. Jonathon Wright cites a study done by researchers treating 20 congestive heart failure patients with far infrared sauna for two weeks on a daily basis. Not surprisingly, 17 of the 20 patients using the FIR sauna showed significant improvement in clinical symptoms, whereas none of the 10 patients in the control group showed any change. The same researchers studied 25 men (ages 31-45) with one or more "coronary risk factors" including diabetes, hypertension, cholesterol, and smoking. These were compared to 10 healthy, younger men (ages 27-43) who did not have these risk factors. Impaired blood vessel dilation was a finding in the risk factor group. **After only two weeks of the daily saunas, the men in the risk factor group showed significant improvements in blood vessel dilation. Naturally, the risk for cardiovascular disease diminished accordingly.**

Before we depart from this discussion on circulation, I invite you to expand your brain's (and body's) circulation a bit more by exposing you to a slightly different train of thought. I mentioned earlier, a sauna or sweat-producing exercise would stimulate your brain, which you may feel you need right about now as you consider this "new" information. For just a moment, tune out of the realm of Newtonian physics' oriented world of physical, tangible Western medicine since what I want to offer is accepted by ancient (and contemporary) Eastern sages, but still not as accepted by most scientists' standards.

There is another type of circulatory system that runs parallel to and is intertwined with the vascular circulatory system in our bodies. I'm not referring to the all-too-important lymphatic system—the body's filtration system which is *not* directly related to the heart. This, as you probably know, moves clear lymphatic fluid through the body. I refer to the vast network that Chinese medicine labels the *meridian system*. This is a structural network of very fine tubular canals, a ductular system that runs along pathways that follow the classical Chinese acupuncture meridians. These microscopic canals not only flow along with and are intertwined in the vascular and lymphatic systems, going in and out of these as proven by radioisotope studies, they form the interface between the protective bioenergetic field some call the *aura* and the deep visceral organs of the body, carrying universal energy into the body. The aura is not acknowledged, as yet, by Western medicine. We'll discuss what's being described here further in the section on electrical fields. Before you judge this as New Age hype if you're unfamiliar with it, remember that no one really understands what electricity is. We can't see it, but we can measure it. We learned how to harness and use it to improve our lives. Science has proven we have bioelectric bodies. And, what Western medicine terms "connective tissue" is really another non-visible circulatory system of pathways.

There is an encapsulating, interfacing, protective energy layer called *wei chi*, or protective chi, in Chinese medicine. I describe this in much greater detail in my up-coming book on Qigong. This chi interfaces with the body's (believed to be roughly 72,000 or so) chakra-linked energy threads, or *nadis*, as called by Indians in their ayurvedic healing system, and would probably correspond to what is (discredited by mainstream) the auric field. Most Western scientists have yet to accept the valid existence of this system. Why? Because one cannot dissect this on a cadaver or living person. Therefore, since you can't see it, naturally, it does not exist! (So, I suppose, neither does electricity.)

The first evidence of this was demonstrated by Dr. Kim Bong Han in the 1960s in an experiment using P32 (a phosphorous radioisotope). When P32 was injected into an acupuncture point, it followed the path of the meridian (energy flow pathway) described in ancient tests, right up to its target organ. There are over 600 of these points located in particular areas of the body. Pierre de Vernejoul further confirmed this using radioactive technetium (99m). In four to six minutes, the dye traveled a distance of 30cm. What's really fascinating is that this system, superimposed along the vascular and lymphatic systems, ends its long road in the tissue cell nuclei—the actual DNA-containing command center of the cell of the particular organ system it is related to. The yellow brick road leads straight to the heart of the Emerald City, so-to-speak. The seemingly unbelievable implication of this is that with the right instrumentation in the field of nanotechnology currently being developed, ultra fine probes (one-billionth of a meter) will be able to deliver microdoses of a drug right into the heart of a very cell that is unhealthy!

A non-visible system runs along a visible system that connects with the external energies and are picked up by the body via acupuncture points—kind of like bioenergetic entrance ramps on these vast, non-visible pathways. It interacts with the internal chemistry of the body, follows a non-visible path along its main circulatory conduits and has been described not only by those such as Dr. Richard Gerber in "Vibrational Medicine," but also ancient spiritual sages, to carry with the body fluids, everything the circulatory and lymphatic system carries, and in much greater quantities. This is amazing when you think about it. Studies show that the amounts of chemical messengers, endocrine system secretions, hyaluronic acid, hormones, steroids, etc., were more than doubled in this system. Physical destruction (surgical cutting) was shown to disrupt this independent energy system. Negative emotions—what the Chinese termed the Seven Demons,

were also shown to retard or block altogether, the nutrient and energy flow known as chi in the system, which leads to malfunction and
ultimate deterioration of the end-target organ associated with the particular meridian in a very short time. Specific emotions damage corresponding organs. Louise Hay of Hay House publishing and radio program-
ming fame, assisted in her own cancer cure which led to her writing an
excellent book entitled, *"You Can Heal Your Life,"* based on linking specific emotions and beliefs to specific organs and medical conditions.

This meridian system has been described as the bioenergy template
for the formation of actual anatomical organs, and may very well be
the missing link that provides answers to puzzling medical mysteries
that surround a disease. An organ's origin has been explained by
Eastern sages as appearing right after conception, and verified bioenergetically by researchers, to have been formed in less than a day after
fertilization. Each of these meridians resonate with a specific, measurable bioelectrical frequency. I use these frequencies to regulate a
meridian's imbalanced energy to restore balance as treatment for various conditions. Working with this energy is considered the new paradigm of health (new rediscovering old, that is) and termed "vibrational medicine." When vibrational energy ends, life ceases. Ancient
monks and sages, without the benefit of science, laid out in theory and
practice, what modern medicine is just beginning to validate.

Why, you may ask, do I bring this "new age" type of medical model
into this book—especially if standard medicine has yet to verify, so
thereby refutes it as something to heed? You may even wonder what it
has to do with your need to Know Sweat. Heat, as I said, has an expansive effect on matter. Bodily components such as blood, lymph fluid,
and other fluids are certain forms of matter. By virtue of the properties of physics, the expansive property of heat increases the vibrational frequency of molecules, including bio-molecules, and sends

them through the body more readily and rapidly via the volume expansion. Remember, heat actually opens up circulatory vessels, including the lymphatics. Is it not conceivable that it does the same to this microscopic circulatory system, along with the chi that flows, as well? I believe that under everyday conditions, particles of disease in the form of stray cancer cells, toxins, sludge—all fine enough to travel through the body—also travel through this non-visible system and carry to areas of the body, the original disease that often bewilders doctors (even those possessed of colossal thinking patterns).

If you think this is absurd, research shows that there are viruses actually living inside of bacteria (once considered the smallest microorganism). When bacteria are killed off (i.e., via antibiotics), the viruses are sometimes released into the body. God only knows what, one day, may be found living in viruses.

These cells may become trapped in an area of bioenergetic constriction and create or initiate the disease right then and there. Heat therapy, although not thoroughly studied on the meridian system per se, as yet, probably has the pattern of breaking up areas of stagnation, including the potential end-result of disease-causing energy, by accelerating the flow of matter and chi through these pathways, even if due to an emotional imbalance believed to be the root cause of a disease. The Chinese made a correlation between stagnated chi and disease. I intend to pursue research on the effects of heat therapy along the meridians.

I've always insisted that energy blockages exist as abnormal vibrational energy wavelengths at the frequency level that permits them to manifest in the body long before any visible manifestation of disease is observed, even using the most high-tech instruments. A dangerous period of time can pass before any medical test shows even the primordial molecular seeds of a disease. This is why this old-turned-new paradigm is so important in my and others' opinion.

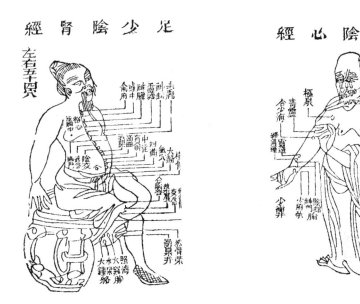

Thus, heat is not just a coincidental benefit or by-product of doing
time-tested mind-body-spirit exercises such as qigong and tai chi by
virtue of expanding life fluids and, thus, energy through not only the
classically accepted circulatory system, but also through this still yet
to be scientifically studied non-visible meridian system in what I
believe to be a pulsatile (passively resonating with, but not dependent
on the pulse). Instead, the amount of heat internally generated by the
frictional resistance of these fluids passing through this mostly unde-
fined system and the interaction (positive and negative) of the blood's
crystalline salts, ions, and other organic and inorganic substances,
may actually be the measure of its chi.

Since these meridians' energy flow patterns are maximized at two-
hour cycles during various times of the day, alternating from system to
system, bioenergetically inducing particular channels to open and
based on assessment of a person's constitutional weakness, this may

maximize flow and clear out blockages. Note that, like certain circadian rhythms related to qigong exercises, it may be difficult to wake up at 2AM to do so. Nevertheless, it's food for thought.

Since it's been shown that energy blockages at this level cause ultimate end-organ failure and disease, and that blockages can also be caused by negative emotions, isn't it conceivable that the emotional feel-good chemicals such as endorphins, dynorphins, and enkephalins have a positive effect on the meridian system and the end organs, possibly "breaking the blues" when they are induced to flow with heat? The implications are astounding.

Immune System Benefits

Sweat therapy, by virtue of physiologic "fever induction," dramatically increases the function of the immune system by activating all of its main defense cells such as neutrophils, macrophages, and T and B lymphocytes (mentioned before) and rushing them to the source of the problem. According to research done by Dr. Wakim and associates at the Mayo Clinic many years ago, numbers of these types of cells which help fight off infections and defend against and combat cancers, increase as much as 58-percent. Their activity levels also increase markedly. *Interferon*, a protein substance that prevents viral reproduction, increases markedly. *Interleukin*, a naturally-occurring immune-response substance, is activated. Protein synthesis changes; and C-reactive protein, which binds to damaged or necrotic cells and some microorganisms, temporarily increases 100-fold. This is a plasma protein sometimes considered an "acute phase protein," which levels rise during inflammatory processes taking place in the body. White blood cell counts increase dramatically. Chronic elevations of these proteins are detrimental to health. Serum, zinc, and iron levels temporarily decrease. *This deprives critical growth factors to invading microorganisms. You stop them dead in their tracks!*

In addition, a recently discovered product of fevers and fever-inducing therapy called *heat shock proteins* is being studied in great detail. Heat shock proteins (HSPs) are also known as stress proteins. These are proteins that are found in all cells in all life forms when a cell experiences different types of environmental stressors such as cold and oxygen deprivation, but mainly in elevated temperatures. They are also present in normal conditions and act as chaperones that make certain a cell's proteins are in the right shape and right place at the right time. Any kind of stress, including disease, causes regular cell proteins to get strung out. They become "undone" due to the unfolding of their building blocks—amino acids. They can help new or distorted proteins get into shape. They also move proteins from one area to another inside the cell, as well as move old proteins into the cell's waste removal system, or recycle bin.

It is believed that HSPs also serve in the presentation of bits of proteins (or *peptides*) on cell surfaces so the immune system notices any diseased cells that need to be taken care of. Research indicates that within cells, heat shock proteins hand over peptides to a different group of molecules. These peptides include normal, as well as abnormal, potential disease-causing proteins. These proteins have been seen to increase in cancers, infectious states, and other disease states of the body. You now know, through the information provided in this book so far, that it's possible to activate them before any disease takes hold. All you have to do is Know Sweat.

Basically the process involves the removal of the abnormal peptides to outside of the cell where the immune system is triggered into action. This research is being used to target and attack different cancers and particular infectious agents. The numbers of these unique proteins increase dramatically with heat therapy. The main classes, which include the small ones (SHSPs), HSP 40, HSP 60, HSP 70, HSP 90, and HSP 100, all have chaperone activity. There are other variants, as well. The HSP 100 variety seems to have the greatest degree of thermo (heat) tolerance. HSPs play an important role in the cell cycle and cancer progression. They help elicit a powerful immune response and are natural immune system boosters.

These proteins have been shown to be a "second arm" of the immune system, led by T cells. The T cells' job, ideally, is to hone in on infected cells (i.e., AIDS) or cancer cells, and destroy them. These are called the CTLs, or *Cytotoxic T cells*. Look at them as the body's internal bouncer removing a drunken, rowdy patron from a bar! There is currently a ton of research going on to integrate specific heat shock proteins into a vaccine form, promoting interest in cancer vaccinations or AIDS vaccinations. It's one of the most exciting immune system subjects being studied today. In the meantime, while you're waiting, create your own vaccination form by stepping into a sauna or steam bath now!

Sweat therapy is beginning to be implemented in the U.S., though it's been used for centuries in clinics around the world. It is now being considered additional therapy for autoimmune diseases, infectious diseases such as hepatitis, rhinoviruses, syphilis, gonorrhea, Epstein-Barr virus, AIDS, and even cancers. And, there is good reason for this. **The Journal of the American Medical Association (JAMA, Vol. 284) states, "Things like unnecessary surgery, medical errors, negative effects of drugs, etc., cause almost as many deaths as heart disease and cancer."** There has to be a better and less potentially harmful way to treat illness.

While sweat therapy may not be a first-line antibacterial or antiviral agent, it should play an important part along with nutrition, Chinese and ayurvedic herbs, homeopathic medicine, and other medical treatment modalities. Hyperthermia, while possibly not capable of killing off every invading organism, can significantly reduce their numbers to a point where the immune system can take care of the rest.

We can see that a real benefit of heat for our body is that we literally burn the enemy out with it. **Many invasive microorganisms can live only in a highly narrow range of temperature. Most begin to die off at about 104°-105°F.** Although they have developed elaborate means of getting into our bodies through the skin, mouth, nose, sex organs, etc., they still have their weaknesses. Most disease-causing bacteria are known as *anaerobes*, in contrast to friendly oxygen-loving *aerobic* bacteria. This means they do not thrive in higher pH, oxygen-rich environments. It is in oxygen-poor, acid-rich environments where their do their dirty work. The use of oxidative therapies (high-oxygen-producing therapies) manages to kill off a good percentage of these microorganisms. They have not yet developed the evolutionary adaptation mechanism to allow them to live in oxygen-rich environments. Thank God! Think of H.G. Wells' *"War of the Worlds"* creatures that were doomed by Earth's microorganisms their own physiology was ill-equipped to cope with.

And, don't think diseases of the body are separate entities as classic medieval textbooks used to call them. Presence of these microorganisms such as bacteria, viruses, fungi, as well as classes that haven't been developed or labeled yet, play a large role in the mix of sludge that when acidified by their nasty secretions, deposit toxins into our heart, brain, kidneys, circulatory vessels, joints, and other areas. Streptococcus is but one example.

I personally believe that much of the disease found in the body is due to lifestyle. Degenerative ailments would not be possible without the presence of such toxin-producing microorganisms and parasites. Even conditions such as arthritis are affected by these. Lifestyle inclusion of yoga, tai chi, qigong, and other sweat-producing, immune system-boosting, mind-body-spirit practices and exercises, along with oxygenating foods and drinks would act as enemies of such microorganisms. As said earlier, sweat therapy and exercise raise the oxygen levels in the body dramatically. Increase in oxygen and heat provides needed fuel for our immune system to burn out many invaders.

As a college student, I played guitar and bass guitar with a band on weekends—not to mention, a pretty decent fiddle. Among the different styles of music we played, one piece we played ad nauseam at Italian functions was the Tarantella. Once started, it seemed it would never end. Why, I asked, does this crazy piece of music with only minor variation, get played on and on? Later, I learned this dance originated in a town called Taranta in the mountains of Italy. There, it was danced day and night, over and over. How this ties in with sweat therapy is that a spider that is a close cousin to the tarantula spider, cohabits with humans in these hot areas. The spider's painful bite and toxin causes victims to get sick and sometimes die. Since anti-venom was not available in earlier times, the way to treat those bit was to get them to dance to this never-ending repetitive piece of music in an attempt to induce fever and sweat the toxin out. Pretty clever how social and cultural aspects serve a healing process.

Okay, what about cancer? Every year, 1.5 million Americans are diagnosed with this disease. I wonder how many cases are missed? It is estimated that cancer will surpass heart disease as the number one cause of death in the U.S. in the next few years. Over $200 billion has been spent since 1971 in an attempt to prevent and cure cancer; yet, our chance of developing some form of it is higher than ever. According to *Forbes Magazine*, we are losing the "war on cancer." Despite some pockets of progress noted lately, statistics indicate that the probability is that one in every two men and one in every three women will develop it. The unfortunate and, once again, material side to this is exemplified in an article noted in *The Associated Press*, "Drug companies are seeing that cancer can be lucrative—a multi-billion dollar business." How sad.

Another interesting article in the science section of the *New York Times* (Tues., Sept. 19, 2006) entitled, "The Tumor That Isn't: Blocking a Path to Cancer," stated moles which turn into cancers, i.e., which then turn into malignant melanomas in the skin, for some "unknown" reason just stop growing and become non-cancerous. The same was found in prostates in men. That a malignant tumor with a mutated gene—a gene that lets the tumor proliferate wildly—just turns itself off in different parts of the body and becomes non-cancerous, defies many of the theories behind this dreaded disease.

Is it possible that we can give this process a (destructive) boost with heat therapy? Hmmm... As I have often said, "Heat is the enemy of disease." Many scientists have said that the majority of cancers, which I believe are actually a form of progressive degenerative disease, could be prevented by lifestyle and dietary change. Couple that with heat therapy, and I think we have a fighting chance. Here's something to think about:

Direct killing of cancer cells begins to occur when cancerous tissue reaches about 104°-105.8°F. This was stated by Dr. M. Dewhirst, Professor of Radiation Oncology and Director of the Duke Hyperthermia Program at the Duke University Medical Center, Durham, NC.

Cancer, by the way, like many other diseases, is simply the end-product of a system overwhelmed by toxicity. Toxic foods, emotions, and lifestyles can cause cancer. The immune system can fight off toxicity for just so long. At some moment in time, the toxicity inundates the body and we see the tipping point. Free radicals—destructive, charged particles which result from a weakened immune system—take command of your weakest constitutional organ system and cause aberrant cell division which turns on the switch for the dormant genes of the disease; but, unfortunately, not the destruction of these aberrant cells once these cells divide. They are, simply defined, unstable molecules with an unpaired electron that steals an electron from another molecule, causing harm to the body. They are among the main culprits which lower oxygen levels and promote an acidic environment in the body—two conditions that are precursors for the formation of cancer and other degenerative diseases. Their damage is perhaps most visibly noticed in oxygen-rich organs such as the brain, liver, heart, kidneys, lungs, and eyes. At the most primordial level, they not only damage the cell membrane and all connective tissue, but notably the cells' DNA, nucleic acid, and mitochondria. These are components of the division-regulating command center of a cell. Accelerated, faulty, aberrant, and unrestrained cell growth now takes place, producing cells with a greatly extended, seemingly immortal life span. These cells just do not seem to want to die, as in the programmed death of normal cells. In general, the tumor, from a bioenergetic perspective, originates wherever your weakest bioelectrical organ system is—where chi (life energy) flow or chakra-based (energy center) energy is weakest. (Another good reason to practice energy-moving, wave-form-producing, chi-boosting qigong exercises.) Hint: When you look at the structure of DNA, a double helix wave-shaped form, you begin to see the subtle correlation between this energy and physical structure. DNA is actually morphologically a wave, coiled into a spiral so that the maximum amount of information can be represented in the least amount of space.

Cell division takes place every second in the body. It is the biological basis for life. Nevertheless, these divisions take place billions of times on a daily basis, usually without a problem, along with millions of cancerous cell divisions occurring and being overwhelmed by good cells.

However, at the most basic vibrational energy or bio-frequency level measured in wavelengths, the toxicity affects the metabolic processes inside the cell, especially in the DNA, damaging the structure of its double helix. And, yes, negative emotions have a negative bio-frequency, as well!

It is estimated that between 1,000-1,000,000 molecular lesions per cell per day occur in the human genome (hereditary information); but thanks to the protective tumor suppressor genes, they are overcome by these "guardian angels" of the body. The damage done to the DNA through different toxic mechanisms will cause it to be damaged through the complicated process of oxidation, ankylation, hydrolysis, or just plain bad DNA replication. Once significant DNA damage has occurred, cells start dividing wildly and uncontrollably, and the end-product is the dreaded disease.

Cancers can form the primary mass (tumor), metastasize ("change of state" in Greek), and spread to other sites in the body making disease much more difficult to control since it now saps the body's nutrients and life energy at a highly accelerated level, and releases a much higher degree of life-destroying toxins. The metastatic spread through blood and lymphatic tissue and quite possibly through the meridian ductule system described earlier, often in late stages of cancer, virtually always sends identical cells of the original tumor to other tissues and organs. There is also a tendency for cancers to "seed." This was first discussed by Stephen Paget in his "seed and soil" theory over a century ago. The "seeds" of the cancer cells are often found migrating to the pleural and peritoneal cavity. *It is much easier to kill the seeds with heat therapy than attack a tumor the size of an orange that has already formed its blood vessels and other structural components.* Remember, heat kills cancer cells. Regular "Know Sweat" therapy may very well help the body rid itself of these undesirable cells at their earliest stages, and even in their spreading stage.

Want to see some "scientific medical" confirmation? Look at the April 18, 2006 issue of the *Wall Street Journal*, in an article titled, "Adding Heat to Cancer Therapy," by Laura Johannes. She states that, "Recent

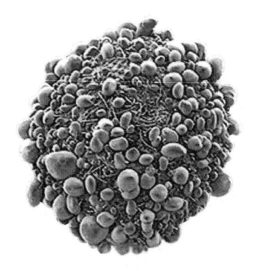

CANCER CELL

studies show that adding hyperthermia, or heat therapy, to traditional radiation and chemotherapy can boost their effectiveness in certain cancers." She adds that in hyperthermia, the cancerous area of the body is heated up to 113°F using various methods including microwave antennas, hot water baths, and infrared lamps. She also said that (italics are mine), **"By itself, heat therapy can kill some cancer cells. But its main advantage, advocates say, is making cancer cells more vulnerable to radiation and chemo [sic]."** How about that one?! In the *Journal of Clinical Oncology* last year, it was reported that scientists at Duke University Medical Center found 68.2-percent of their patients who did radiation plus heat, had tumors disappear entirely vs. 23.5-percent of those who got radiation alone. Hippocrates talked about the ability of heat to eliminate disease long before any one of us was even a spiritual essence in a person's genes—or jeans!

When you detoxify yourself, you may begin to help detoxify cancer cells right out of your body. Certainly better than invasive procedures. A really good detoxifying system for dealing with a condition such as cancer, or any illness or imbalance, works better if it involves mind-body-spirit cooperation.

Referencing, once again, the timeless wisdom of Dr. Paavo Airola, "Cancer is a disease of civilization's living and eating habits, which result in a biochemical imbalance and physical and chemical irritation of the tissues." He cites the research done by Dr. Willar J. Visek of Cornell University, who was one of the pioneers to draw a connection between a high-protein diet and the development of cancer. Ammonia, a product which is produced in high amounts as the by-product of meat metabolism, is noted to be highly carcinogenic and can be at least one factor in the development of cancers. Also cited in Dr. Airola's, "Biological Treatments" section on cancer, is fever therapy.

Getting back to the basics and away from all the DNA dialogue, since ammonia is one of the components of sweat and therapeutic sweating, I think we can now make the argument for getting rid of excess ammonia as a result of sweat therapy. Hospital records show that Seventh Day Adventists, Mormons, and Navajo Indians eat very little or no meat and suffer from cancers far seldom than the average American. I'm not saying cut meat out entirely, but use caution. And, if you do eat meat, eat certified organic or kosher since these are deemed by experts to be the healthiest to consume.

Aside from fasting, oxygen therapies, amalgam and infected tooth removal, adequate rest, spiritual enhancement, nutritional and immune-boosting support, fever therapy is cited as "one of the most effective cancer treatments" used in the famous, late, Dr. Josef Issels' cancer clinic in Germany, as well as in many other biological clinics around the world. Dr. Issels' whole-body therapy protocol, which continues to be used by other doctors, involves strenghtening the entire body versus attacking the tumor. In one study, 370 of Dr. Issels' patients, with various types and stages of cancer, followed his protocol. After five years, 87-percent were still alive and showed no signs of recurrent cancer. A note on cancer and sweat therapy: It takes real effort and patience to get a person with advanced cancer to sweat. It isn't known for certain why this is, though it may tie in with what I said earlier about the shutting down of the body's ability to sweat once the body's immune and other systems are compromised to a certain level—especially if compromised by certain microorganisms.

You may have noticed television commercials that began to air during summer of 2006 for drugs to treat certain cancers caused by viruses. That should make you want to break a sweat! Especially since you now know that heat therapy kills viruses and microorganisms. A definite link has been made between Human Papillomavirus (HPV) and cervical cancers, as well as Epstein-Barr virus—believed to cause mononucleosis and types of lymphomas (lymph node cancers) in Africa. They contribute to a formation of a particularly nasty type of cancer called Burkitt's Lymphoma, the hepatitis virus (and, probably, all variants of this), and hepatomas (liver cancers), as well as many, many others soon to be discovered. These viruses lurk around, usually for long periods of time in their latency period, until something such as your immune system weakening, makes them spring to action to make you sick.

When I say "long periods of time," I really mean a long time. I'm not using this as a religious book to validate the belief of "sins of the fathers" as proposed in biblical text; but, there are (coincidental?)

findings that support the fact that certain diseases such as breast cancer may not be the result of an infection as it is the result of latent viral DNA that may exist in the body and be unknowingly passed on from generation to generation, perhaps, from seven generations before. Such disease may exist silently in the body until a switch is turned on upsetting the immune system in a way that brings on the disease, something for which a lack of risk factors doctors and scientists cannot explain sufficiently. The stressor may be biological, spiritual, emotional, environmental, or any combination. Other examples are the sexually transmitted diseases of syphilis and gonorrhea, as described by Dr. Hahnemann in his *"Theory of Miasms."* Dr. Samuel Hahnemann, father of homeopathy, a practice still largely refuted by our medical system (though Great Britain's royal family is rumored to use homeopathy), described these energies as miasms—the vibrational energy carried by the essence of the disease.

A personal note on cancer and vibrational medicine. Even those who are sick and dying can be influenced, if they allow themselves to be, and brought back to health with the loving effect of compassion, kind and supportive words, and positive thoughts. Prayer, an example of this, has been shown to demonstrate extraordinary benefit, especially when a person is open to receiving it. These positively-charged vibrational energy emotions and thought forms help refract and, thus, negate, bioenergetically, the paralyzing fear generated by the cancer cells' vibrational energy. Projection of such, will actually change the resonant frequency of the patient's molecules in the body while effectively harmonizing and strengthening immune system cells that resonate at much higher frequencies. This, possibly, hampers and refracts the negative frequencies of viruses and cancer cells that are mostly water (like all other cells), which has been shown to retain these frequencies even if for a short period of time. True appreciation, giving thanks, and adopting a life purpose "treatment" approach (finding a higher purpose in life) allows a person to create this body-mind-spirit environment for him- or herself. I've been able to measure the effect of such practice in my clinic, time after time.

If you have reason, scientific or otherwise, to suspect that cancers may have a viral or microbial cause, including parasites and their eggs—and I feel ample scientific proof of this is emerging on a daily basis—isn't it a smart approach to "nip it in the bud" and kill these microorganisms with heat and other lifestyle modifications before they manifest as disease? In Chinese philosophy, there is a quote I refer to often: "Treating disease after it arises is like beginning to dig a well after one has become thirsty..." Use the Zen Warrior Spirit I write about in, *"Zen and the Way of the Sword."* Become the sword to destroy these pathological entities so you can continue to enjoy life. It's brief enough as it is.

Another major category of immune system disorder, characterized by the presence of the HIV virus, is AIDS (Acquired Immune Deficiency Syndrome). The HIV virus is believed to cause this challenging condition. It is temperature-sensitive, as are other viruses, and suffers a greater degree of inactivation and destruction at progressively higher temperatures above 98.6°F. According to clinical laboratory research (H. Weatherburn, "Hyperthermia and AIDS treatment", from the *British Journal of Radiology*), **the HIV virus is 40-percent inactivated by lying in a water bath of 107.6°F for 30 minutes. At 132.8°F, it becomes 100-percent inactive.**

There is still a tremendous debate regarding HIV as the sole or primary cause of AIDS. While most people with AIDS test positive for HIV, and hundreds of thousands of papers have been written on this and billions of dollars spent on research for a "cure," the jury is still out on this one. HIV, which belongs to the retrovirus family, is believed to lead to life-threatening infections. Yet, the virus, itself, is not cytocidal (capable of killing cells). University of California professor of molecular and cell biology, Peter Duesberg, clearly pointed this out in his research on the different presentations of the disease in different geographic and cultural groups, even making the categorization of this disease "a dilemma." What if there is severe immune system compromise in a group—potentially exacerbated by extremely poor lifestyle choices, drug addiction, and other infections—and HIV cannot be found? Then, is it still AIDS?

When researcher Robert Gallo first announced on April 23, 1984, that a new retrovirus, an RNA-containing virus with tumor-causing properties initially called HTLV-III, had been identified as the causative agent of AIDS, it was really based on a hypothesis. The press reports citing HIV as the probable cause of AIDS, were quietly dropped and became cited as "The Cause for AIDS." Therefore, the official standard is that HIV causes AIDS. Don't think so. It's much more complex than that. In any case, there are people who have HIV and never get AIDS. There are also people who have had full-blown AIDS reversed to HIV-negative status, based on documented evidence by a particular doctor using oxygen therapies such as medical ozone therapy. This doctor has, subsequently, been stripped of everything he had, lucky to be alive, and works as a farmer in a rural community.

As complex as this 120 nanometer or 120 billionth of a meter (very, very tiny), nine-gene-containing bizarre-looking organism is, it has its weaknesses. All things do. I say bizarre-looking because it looks like something that came from outside our natural world. Many, including myself, have theories as to its origin, which is highly suspect. It is composed of two copies of positive single-stranded RNA that contain these complex genes, and is enclosed by a conical capsid which is composed of 2,000 copies of the viral protein. Surrounding the capsid is a matrix compound of viral protein. This viral protein is surrounded by two layers of fatty molecules called phospholipids—taken from the membrane of a human cell it attaches to. Although it is an insidious, complex, and constantly mutating virus, it does have its enemies. An extremely high-oxygen environment is one of them. As you may have guessed and I've already explained, a good degree of heat is the other. Heat actually degenerates and decomposes the fatty- and protein-protective coat of this virus.

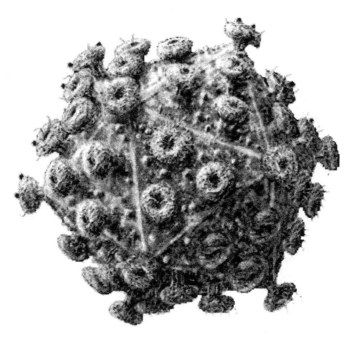

AIDS VIRUS

I know individuals who, when others would have succumbed, used the Zen Warrior Spirit to fight this by using oxygen therapies such as ozone, hyperbaric, and hydrogen peroxide therapies, as well as an enhanced nutrition program that utilizes Chinese and ayurvedic herbs, mind-body-spirit practices, and tons of heat therapy to literally cook this demon right out of their bodies. They now live perfectly healthy lives. If you or someone you love has this disease, tell them not to despair.

Also, do not let others use this condition to promulgate a cowardly, and often judgmental, hypothesis as I've seen done so many times before. There is too much scientific evidence about any disease, including this one, to call any of them "God's punishment." People who do this, do so in order to justify their own practices and belief system. Disease, like all other processes, is simply an imbalance that can, but does not have to, remain a disease. As a dedicated healer, I don't like any disease being used as a political tool. Tell anyone you know who has this disease to follow the steps I outline in this book. Tell them to utilize whatever other means necessary to defeat this disease entity. We are all God's children, even those who do not "live perfectly." In fact, no one lives perfectly. What I'm about to share here is based on my beliefs: I believe we are intended to be happy and to live each day as a great day.

Getting back to the general foundation of health and homeostasis... In the same way the body's metabolism slows down when a person doesn't take in enough calories daily (hopefully, the right kinds of calories), perhaps when a disease is advanced, cells have some intrinsic survival mechanism that exerts an inhibitory mechanism on the body which causes it to resist sweating—much like after a meal, your body focuses on digestion. For all the reasons mentioned to this point, and including scores of others coming to light as this is being written, sweat therapy should play an integral role in cancer and other disease treatment. Heating the body protects and enhances the function of normal cells and makes tumor cells more susceptible to chemotherapy and radiation—should this be the route a person chooses.

Sweat Therapy, Elimination, and Aging-Effects Determent
This section should really be called, "How to Retire Rich by Taking on Some Heat." Sweating out toxic accumulations through your skin,

lessens the load on the liver and, probably more importantly, on the kidneys. You essentially "bypass" these organs, keeping them healthier longer. In this case, "use it or lose it" shouldn't apply. You don't want to over-use these organs! When you do, they simply age faster and sooner than they may have been programmed to. Sweating lightens the workload on these organs by using the largest organ of the body, the skin, for some of the needed elimination. If you increase the efficiency of your circulatory system, especially with heat, you clean out the major organ systems such as the liver, kidneys, lungs, and intestines. As a major component of the gastrointestinal system, the liver is probably the most over-worked organ.

The aging process, accelerated by toxins and free radical attacks, is hampered by the nervous system's healthy circulation process. I said it before and I'll say it again: **Sweating helps you look and feel younger longer**. Unless we actively do something to preserve mental function like mental stimulation, exercise, and sweat therapy, the end result is decreased cerebral (brain) blood flow and decreased numbers of neurons (nerve cells).

Sweat therapy allows us to get longer use out of these organs and potentially live longer and healthier, as well. Think about how long an automobile lasts if it isn't over-driven, uses the right octane fuel for its engine, has its fluids changed (detoxified) on a regular basis, and is allowed to warm up and get the oil into the engine when we first start it up before driving. Proper maintenance of a car increases its performance and longevity—despite the disposable mind-set that seems to permeate much of society. The body operates on the same principle as a car.

Incidentally, scientists constantly try to find ways to slow down the aging process. As far back as the 1930s, researchers stumbled onto a ridiculously simple way to slow down the biological aging forces—cutting back caloric intake by a third. This was shown to increase life span of animals by 30- to 40-percent. Certain researchers applied these principles to themselves. Sure, it's good to eat less, but not at the expense of looking like a clothes hanger wearing a suit. It isn't necessary to appear like a lean anatomy lesson, resembling the figures in the curiously morbid exhibit, "Bodies," to gain health benefits. As I write this, a tour of this name and description is currently making its way around the U.S.

In 1956, a University of Nebraska researcher proposed that "free radicals" cause aging. These are a destructive, reactive oxygen species, as noted before. I think every vitamin company, knowledgeable and ignorant, jumped on this bandwagon. In the 1990s, genetic hypotheses were presented and now (for your intellectual curiosity) it is reported that *resveratrol*, a substance in red wine, has shown to increase the life span of yeast, a very simple microorganism and, just recently did the same for a fish species—as reported by Italian scientists. Before you begin to celebrate this bit of news and seek validation for your love of wine, consider this: You are neither a yeast nor a fish. You would truly need to become a wino to enjoy these benefits. You'd need to drink hundreds of glasses of wine a day to achieve the same results. I feel some wine is good for the cardiovascular and nervous system, on many levels. The key, once again as the Tao reminds us, is moderation.

The liver is always busy performing its 600-plus functions. It is the major detoxifier of all the drugs and alcohol we put into our bodies. The liver breaks down the by-products of endocrine or hormonal secretions and detoxifies other poisons, as well. It not only filters the blood to remove large toxins, it synthesizes and secretes bile which contains cholesterol, a necessary substance, despite all the negative media hype. Bile, unfortunately is a carrier of many toxic substances and must be eliminated through the intestines. Bilirubin, a breakdown product of red blood cells, is in this mix. The liver also disassembles toxic chemical components through the mechanism of oxidation, reduction, and hydrolysis.

This workhorse weighs in at about 1,500 grams. It is susceptible to damage from bacteria, viruses, toxic compounds, and parasites— believed by many to be the root cause of disease (Dr. Hulda Clark). An example of this is damage from the different types of *hepatitis*. People who have hepatitis need to know there are easier and healthier means to manage and even eliminate this degenerative ailment, such as the ones described in this book. It is ironic that we can kill off up to 90-

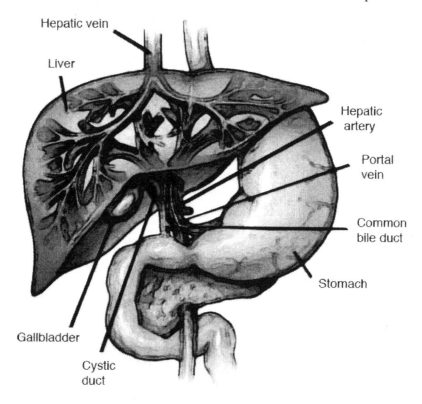

LIVER DIAGRAM

percent of the liver's functional cells, called hepatocytes, and it still continues to serve us like an obedient dog.

Even while it valiantly continues to clean up our body, eventually, an over-stressed or damaged liver will fail to prevent an accumulation of toxicity in our body. The good news is, it doesn't have to go this far.

The liver is an important component of the body's five primary detoxification systems; the others are the respiration, urinary, lymphatic, gastrointestinal—a system of which the liver is a part, and, of course, there is the skin. The liver is also an important component of elimination pathways known as Phase I and Phase II. In the Phase I pathway, enzymes directly neutralize some chemicals, but most are converted to intermediate forms which are then processed in Phase II. The Phase I intermediates, according to world-noted nutritional authority, Dr. Larry Milam, are more chemically active and, therefore, more toxic. If the Phase II systems are not working right, we have the potential to develop serious disease. The Phase I detox involves a group of 50-100 enzymes which are a part of what is called the Cytochrome P450 System. The P450 enzyme system of Phase I is easily disrupted by the substances that will cause excess free radical activity. These range from alcohol, drugs, toxic fumes, pesticides, fats, heavy metals, microorganisms... You name it.

In the Phase II system, called the conjugation pathway, liver cells attempt to dilute a toxin by adding substances such as cysteine, glycerine, or sulfur molecules to make these water-soluble. Remember, both Phase I and Phase II systems diminish in efficiency with age. Therefore, lifestyle improvement, nutritional supplements, and exercise will prolong the efficiency of these pathways. When these pathways have been damaged or compromised from life in our toxic world, what can you count on to take up the slack? Yep, the good old skin, once again. No Sweat?

The kidneys, which work in close conjunction with the liver, are the major eliminators of the body. They not only remove waste, they also function to maintain fluid and electrolyte balance in the body. The kidneys excrete urine via the activity of about two-million nephrons (the kidneys' functional filtration units—about one-million in each kidney). Fluid is filtered from blood and converted to urine as it passes to the renal pelvis. Therefore, metabolic end-products, excess sodium ions, potassium, chloride, and hydrogen, are cleared from the blood plasma. Aside from being our waste-disposal organs, the kidneys dispose of extracellular fluid rich in sodium, chloride, bicarbonate, but low in potassium, magnesium, and phosphates. This is in contrast to intracellular fluid rich in potassium, magnesium, proteins, and inorganic and organic phosphates. This helps the body protect itself against lethal diseases and hypertension by expelling extra water and salt. The ravages of hypertension include coronary artery disease, congestive heart disease, rupture of the brain's blood vessels (hemorrhagic stroke), and kidney failure—the increased pressure destroys the kidneys' own functional elements. When this happens, controlling blood pressure can be next to impossible.

Old Chinese medical texts often refer to vitality as kidney chi. This reproductive essence or *jing*, as it is called, draws attention to the great importance of the kidney-adrenal complex. Other ayurvedic-based healing systems sometimes refer to this as the "kundalini," or coiled serpent-of-life energy in the body. Chinese medicine makes note of the fact that about half of a person's kidney chi is lost by the age of 40. Even if there is a metaphorical significance to this, there is some truth to it. Most of us walk around with at least some sub-clinical or non-detectable degree of kidney impairment, especially when we hit our forties and fifties, primarily from toxic accumulations. Subtle bioenergy changes take place in the body which are almost indiscernible. This may explain why people can live with a single kid-

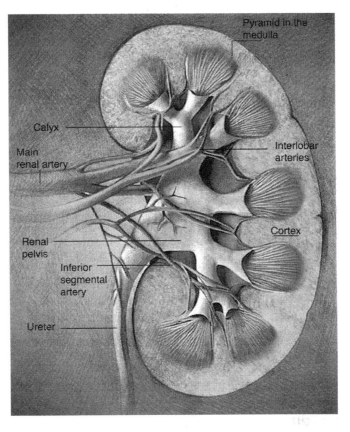

KIDNEY DIAGRAM

ney, such as kidney transplant recipients, and not have problems.

The strep throats we endured as children (and sometimes as adults) introduced us to the culprit bacteria known as *streptococcus* that produces an endotoxin that damages not only the heart's valves, the body's joints, the brain and other organs, but the kidneys' tubules, as well. Add to this high salt and cholesterol levels of the Western diet, metabolic by-products of medicines (antibiotics, pain medications, recreational and non-recreational drugs, and others), pesticides, environmental pollutants, food overload, and heavy-metal toxins—to mention a few—and this means it is possible that we may have finished off many more of these nephrons than we thought. We may be walking around with a loss of 50-percent of the nephrons we started out with. In Chinese medicine, that's a loss of 50-percent of chi (life energy); but, the kidneys have a unique way of compensating for any loss. The remaining nephrons become hypertrophied (get larger) and become more active. Blood tests such as BUN (blood-urea-nitrogen) that measure kidney function and creatinine, appear to be normal even at this stage. We don't even know anything is wrong. We are tricked into believing all is okay. This is what makes it possible to live a normal life with one well-functioning kidney.

Since streptococcus occurs in the mouth area, mouth bacteria may one day be implicated in many of today's diseases. In fact, it already is. It was mentioned previously that many microorganisms cannot live in an oxygen-rich environment. Once the mouth is in a poor-oxygen condition caused by smoking, dryness, etc., mouth germs can rapidly propagate. There is significant evidence that when there are problems in the body, there are problems in the mouth. Since these readily migrate into the blood when there is a diminished resistance such as in periodontal disease, which affects an estimated 87-percent of Americans to some degree or another, they settle in heart valves, kidneys, joints, the brain, placenta of pregnant women—and cause different diseases in these areas. Links have been made between certain dental conditions and prostate cancer. The mouth is the gate-keeper, in many ways, of the body. Take SweetKiss™ daily (www.lef.org/800.544.4440).

Practice good sense about better overall hygiene. It isn't necessary to become compulsive about washing our hands every time we touch something. Unless our immune systems are compromised, our natural defense mechanisms are equipped to handle a lot of the microorganisms we come in contact with every day. Here's one hygienic practice that should be embraced. Years back, a report stated every time a toilet is flushed, particulate matter is dispersed up to about six feet into the air. How many of you leave your toothbrush out and your toilet lid up? I note a correlation between dental and overall health in various sections of this book. This is one situation where it's best to keep a lid on it. Close the toilet cover before you flush!

From a non-medical, metaphorical perspective, leaving the toilet seat up and open is not just an ongoing conflict between men and women. In Feng Shui, this signifies "drainage" or dissipation of wealth—going down the tube (or toilet) so-to-speak. Along with wealth, down does the life energy of the home. So, energetically speaking, think of what you're letting in and what is draining out. Keeping the toilet closed when not in use, can not only change the energy in your home, but save a relationship. Ask any man who's been the recipient of a woman's ire if she's surprised by "taking a swim" when nature calls in the middle of the night.

Back to the kidneys. Nephrons don't regenerate. If the loss of nephrons progresses, we begin to see the signs. Azotemia (increased nitrogen concentration), frequent urination, decreased ability to break down proteins, impaired urine concentration, and perhaps even back pain happens. Chinese medicine refers to back pain as chi depletion. But even if these things occur, it's still not that serious. At 75-percent nephron loss, we actually begin to see signs of renal insufficiency. If this progresses, things do get worse. At this stage, welcome to the wonderful world of allopathic medicine which may include dialysis to clear waste products from your body. It seems it would be a lot easier if we chose to deliberately sweat long before we allow end-stage renal disease (ESRD) to happen. Use your common sense with the wisdom I'm giving you. It's not too late to begin sweat therapy regimens.

Strengthen and maintain what you have left. Don't drive on the already-worn spare tire. There is no other in your trunk. You can create your own at-home, do-it-yourself "dialysis" and never create the need for the allopathic version.

It was pointed out by Aaland (1997) that **a 15-minute sauna session is capable of eliminating the same amount of toxic waste, such as urea and uric acid, as the kidneys would normally take 24 hours to perform. A whole day of detox in 15 minutes**. How's that for efficiency?!

If someone you know is undergoing dialysis, the "fat lady" hasn't sung yet; so, don't throw in the towel. It would still be beneficial for them to sweat—of course, under the supervision of a knowledgeable health care provider or doctor. It would help them not need as much dialysis and would increase the life span and quality of life.

Going back to the first sentence of this section, your health is your wealth. When you've protected this aspect of your life (like your monetary investments) and enhanced it, you will more than likely get to enjoy and savor your retirement and all the wonderful accoutrements that go along with it. I've known multi-millionaires to lose it all by losing their health and, perhaps, life. Money without health cannot be enjoyed. Maybe enjoyed by someone else, but not by you. In my many years in health care, ministerial work, and other forms of spiritually-enhancing practices, I've never come across a person who took anything material with them when they died. No chariot transports tangibles to the promised land. Bring on the heat and better lifestyle. Then, when it's time to go, at least you know you've given it your all and, hopefully, with a smile on your face.

Sweat Therapy and Detoxification
As we forge ahead and enjoy great technological gains, we also see there is a price attached to this that comes in the form of pollution and

destruction of resources, primarily because industry moguls don't focus on cleaner means or potential short- or long-term negative impacts. In the sad story, *"The Lorax,"* the greed and wantonly destructive ways of the human race are poignantly depicted in the teachings of one of my favorite, and beloved by many, old-time authors Theodor Seuss Geisel, known simply as Dr. Seuss.

This story was brought to life in a musical play I helped produce for my son's third grade class, presented to his school. The memory still brings tears of joy! In this tale, Dr. Seuss' most controversial one, the plight of the environment is chronicled. The Lorax—a mossy, bossy man-like creature—speaks for the trees against the greedy Once-ler, and tells a boy about a beautiful sunny forest full of truffula trees that was devastated by the Once-ler's heedless cutting down and harvesting of these trees, thus, polluting the environment and darkening the sky. It becomes accelerated (accelerated need for corporate profits) until there is but one truffula seed left between the beautiful tree's extinction and continuity; and it will become extinct unless... The story ends with this message. Perhaps non-jaded nine-year-olds still understand what the rest of humanity is missing. We will poison our environment and our bodies unless...

Also, because most of us no longer grow or raise our own food sources, we are dependent on what others provide for us. What we ingest is, more than likely, affected by some level of contamination. Some foods are irradiated. Irradiation causes toxic substances in the foods such as benzene and formaldehyde to be formed.

Something else most people are unaware of is we ingest about 210 micrograms of phthalates per day. Phthalates are used to soften plastics, including the ones used by the medical industry, as well as solvent agents in cosmetics and other products. Phthalates are known to cause damage to the liver, kidneys, lungs, and reproductive organs.

They out-gas from virtually every plastic material including wraps, Styrofoam, etc. This is magnified when they are used to cover food in a microwave oven. They can damage DNA and disrupt the endocrine and other systems. The result is premature aging and disease. A by-product of plastic is styrene. Styrene is notorious as a cancer producer in humans. Dr. Sherry Rogers cites that styrene is found in 100-percent of all fat tissues sampled in biopsies. This means that **every one of us has this poison stored in our fat cells waiting for a moment to wreak havoc.** But, don't panic. Sweat, detox, and use as few plastic products as possible. New threats include the gasoline additive MTBE, volatile organic compounds, new pesticides, and other aberrational forwards the public has not yet heard of—over 4,000 of them, to be precise.

By the way, if you're thinking of moving to some remote island paradise in the South Pacific or a small town to get away from it all, *fugeddaboudit*. Studies have shown that circulating convection currents in the air carry the most poisonous toxic waste from industrial centers and dump them on rural towns hundreds of miles away, causing a bewildering array of diseases people, at one time, could not link to any natural causes—until, of course, meteorologists explained the line. As I said before, you can run, but you can't hide, as the expression goes. The pollution of our world is not going to go away anytime soon. Now would be a good time to take a stand if you haven't already. One way you can do your part is to become involved with preventing the massive deforestation of areas such as the Amazon (a pharmacologically-rich environment) and become involved with the movement to stop global warming and pollution. Hopefully, it's not too late—but, it really is getting worse.

I want to make a disclaimer now, since the information I'm providing here seems so negative: Our bodies are designed to battle and eliminate invaders, and thus protect us—up to a certain point, of course. Just as I mentioned what's needed to keep an automobile running at maximum efficiency, we are able to keep the balance with some fairly simple techniques—sweat therapy being a primary one. As you continue to read this information, remember you are not a victim in this matter. Our bodies are equipped to cope with and manage certain levels of invasive hitch-hikers. We have problems when the toxic accumulations spill over like a glass over-filled with liquid. The purpose of this book is not to act like Chicken Little and cry out that "the sky is falling." It is to empower you with information so you have more of what you want—health and quality of life—than what you don't want. That said, I'll continue.

Heavy metals such as mercury, cadmium, aluminum, antimony, and arsenic are found in our environment because of waste products that are discarded ineffectively. Even though it's still denied by some in the field, the link between aluminum toxicity and Alzheimer's disease has been pretty much recognized. Arsenic, known as a poison, is sometimes used in root canals. Ironically, some of the ancient religious scriptures note its efficiency in treatment of disease from infections, possibly even cancers. Hair dyes contain levels of lead we want to be aware of. These metals and other substances work their way into our food sources, our bodies, and even mother's milk. You may not be able to completely eliminate them, but you can reduce their levels and subsequent effects on your body. A fact: When smokers finish using a public sauna, a brownish tar and nicotine residue is often left behind to be cleaned from the benches.

Here's something noteworthy and of interest. A very dear friend of mine, Jim Woodworth, a man with a heart of platinum—not gold, has established the most comprehensive detox protocol for firefighters, policemen, and other persons affected by the tragic destruction of the

World Trade Center on September 11, 2001. At the core of his detoxification program is a nutritionally-based sweat therapy protocol, principles which were advocated by L. Ron Hubbard, the famous Scientologist. No matter personal opinions about Scientology, Jim's success ratio is astounding. Towels from patients treated, reflect the poisons coming out of their bodies by emerging as a (toxic) rainbow of colors—another great testament to sweat therapy, the core of his detox regimen at the New York Center for Detoxification (http://nydetox.org/). He has, at the time of this writing, treated over 500 persons successfully. His unselfish humanitarian dedication helped some of those who are most dear to me. What's most striking, is that this project is done with his own financing, along with some voluntary contributions. If you think all of this is bull, take time to read two highly informative books written by L. Ron Hubbard: *"Clear Body, Clear Mind"* and *"Purification: An Illustrated Answer to Drugs."* In my opinion, Hubbard was clearly another one ahead of his time.

The nervous system has a self-defeating mechanism called the *blood-brain barrier*. I mentioned this before, and now will explain it. This is a one-way gate—like a Chinese finger trap. If you're unfamiliar with this amusing trap, it's made of straw. When you put a finger from each hand into the ends and pull, the straw weave tightens and you are unable to remove your fingers. You have to relax any tension and use at least one other finger to hold it in place while you remove the stuck fingers. It's truly a metaphysical symbol that demonstrates the importance of releasing whatever makes you tense. Back to the nervous system. This system allows the entry of various beneficial elements into brain tissue, yet once certain toxins, especially heavy metals, enter the central nervous system, they do not diffuse out again unless we make them do so. By some mechanism yet to be explained, they remain lodged.

This is especially tragic when it comes to children's health. Medical experts are beginning to point out a link between the syndrome called

Autism and heavy metal poisoning. This may be, at the very least, a contributing factor to the development of this awful syndrome. Some experts feel the link is too strong to ignore. Whether this is later proved to be correct (or not), we still need to address the concern generated by increased levels of mercury and other metals in our bodies, and their potential short- and long-term impacts on health.

Autism is characterized by impairments in social interaction, repetitive behaviors, communication, sensory dysfunction, and abnormal movements. Recent epidemiologic studies suggest that it may affect 1 in 150 children in the U.S. If true, that should be just plain unacceptable! I have seen communities in the U.S. where its prevalence appears to be staggeringly higher.

According to a study by S. Bernard, A. Enayati, L. Redwood, H. Roger, and T. Binstock, U.S. government data suggest that

1. Many cases of Idiopathic Autism are induced by mercury exposure from *thimerosol*, a mercury preservative added to many vaccines, and that

2. This type of Autism represents an unrecognized mercurial syndrome; and, that genetic and non-genetic factors establish a predisposition whereby the overall adverse effects occur only in some children. The questionable fact remains, why is this being used in the first place? Has anyone explored the cumulative risks of the preservatives placed in the vaccines?

Here's something you may not be aware of. The expansion of the vaccine market is no longer being limited to children. The vaccine industry has found a whole new target audience—teenagers. These are being advertised and promoted by doctors all over the country. According to the *Wall Street Journal* (Wed., August 23, 2006), drug companies are rolling out vaccines for diseases teenagers may be "at risk" for catching—meningitis, whooping cough, and human papillomavirus virus.

Can a person really *catch* a disease? I would like someone to explain this one to me. I still don't understand it. We certainly can develop a disease if our immune system weakens.

Want to know what else is in those innocuous vaccines your children with undeveloped immune systems are being subjected to? (Note: Innocuous—Inoculation. See the highly suggestive mode of hypnosis?) Dr. Jon Barron, a well-known alternative health physician, lists six major health-destroying elements in his newsletter of 2004. They are

1. *Ethylene glycol* — Otherwise known as antifreeze. Fine for your car's radiator, but certainly not in your child's vaccine.

2. *Phenol* (or carbonic acid) — Used as a disinfectant and dye (a toxic substance).

3. *Formaldehyde* — A cancer-causing agent often used as a preservative, in embalming of the deceased, and sometimes added to tobacco for many cigarette brands sold to the public. (The annoying odor of this chemical permeated our bodies and clothing in the first year of human dissection when I was studying human anatomy. It's still imprinted in my brain's olfactory cortex.)

4. *Aluminum* — Used in vaccines to promote antibody response. Aluminum causes cancer in mice and is associated with seizures and, as most people know by now, Alzheimer's Disease.

5. *Neomycin* and *Streptomycin* — Antibiotics which trigger allergic reactions in some people and, of course, thimerosol, mentioned earlier.

Studies of Autism show that in most affected children, the developmental timing of autistic symptoms coincide with the period corresponding to the administration of the vaccinations. The causal relationship is too great to ignore. Dr. Ronald Miller, a surgeon at the University of Washington Medical Center noted, "Autism was discovered in 1943, in American children twelve years after ethyl mercury (thimerosol) was added to the pertussis vaccine." The disease began to show up in Europe in the 1950s, after the vaccine was introduced there.

Even the FDA and AAP related that the amount of mercury given to infants from vaccinations has exceeded safety levels. According to data published by the Institute for Vaccine Safety at the Johns Hopkins Bloomberg School of Public Health, three varieties of the 2006/2007 influenza vaccines contain thimerosol. Mercury, a potent toxin, makes up 50-percent of thimerosol. A flu shot given to a 20-pound child contains 12.5 micrograms of mercury. This is 14 times the daily amount considered safe by the EPA. A second shot is routinely given a month later. When this is coupled with pre-natal load from mercury amalgams (if the mother has these in her mouth), immune globulin injections, mercury from consumption of fish caught in polluted waters and, of course, our own environmental exposure, a stage for tragedy for the next generation is set up.

I am not giving you a recommendation of whether or not you or your children should or should not take vaccines. Only you can make this choice, and it should be based on your informed-choice, weighing what doctors often cite as the "risk/reward ratio."

My good friend Bill Johnson, owner of High Tech Health International and maker of far infrared saunas, strongly recommends FIR therapy along with other health modifications to, perhaps, undo some of the toxic damage we experience before it becomes totally permanent. He has forwarded to me, letters tearfully written by mothers who describe their child's reversal of this tragic syndrome after use of the far infrared sauna. (High Tech Health International — 1.800.794.5355/www.hightechhealth.com). I'm taking this a step further by combining this amazing treatment with a series of oxygen therapies and nutritional detoxification protocols that have the potential to actually reverse a great deal of the damage in the developing, but still amenable-to-repair infant's nervous system. **A precautionary measure is to do a thorough detox, including sweat therapy, along with nutritionally-based protocols before conception.** I believe this will bring the risks down dramatically.

In my opinion, there is probably some predisposition of the newly developing fetus to be harmed by toxins in a manner never seen before. The new cells in the fetus seem weaker now than at any time in history because of the toxins picked up not only by the mother, but also by the father in terms of internal and environmental toxins, including bioenergetically destructive fields such as cell phones and other electronic instruments despite "findings" reported in 2006 that these are perfectly safe to use. These create holes or perforations in the bioenergetic templates (energy matrix) that surround and permeate the developing embryo. Thus, the energetic anatomy that will dictate the functional anatomy to be formed has already been harmed with breaks in the energy field (aura), and creates stagnant pools of energy in the developing cells as early as the first several divisions. Couple this with our high-stress living, including suppressed emotional influence transmitted by the mother and, perhaps, indirectly by the father, and the infant's protective energy field (wei chi) becomes damaged along with the parents'.

This continues through development and is influenced by shifts in bioenergy patterns every month. Each lunar month affects a developing predominant meridian's bioenergy system. When this happens, the protective energy of the infant is compromised. Detailed conversations with my patients who have children with differing problems have allowed me to validate what the Eastern sages knew—that specific emotional imbalances, especially from the mother at an exact developmental stage (i.e., 2 months, 3 months), can cause problems in associated organ systems, bioenergetically related to the problem in that emotion (i.e., children with liver problems caused by anger or rage, heart defects caused by rejection and sorrow). A preponderance or cascade of these negative emotions at the particular time when the specific organ system is most fragile or vulnerable, can have disastrous results that can last a lifetime. The over-burdened, fragile system is now much more prone to damage from toxic overload—by any means. The toxic hump-breaking straw, in my opinion, is often the vaccine.

Expectant fathers can heed this: Make every attempt not to aggravate the mother of your child while she's pregnant. If you get angry or resentful, find a productive way to communicate feelings and needs that help both of you (and your developing child) benefit. Expectant mothers: Granted, you have hormones flooding your body like never before, but also seek to manage whatever comes up in ways that protect the child you carry in your body. Expectant mothers would benefit greatly by doing some de-stressing activities like listening to soothing music, walks in nature, or meditation. Gentle, non-stressing forms of qigong exercises are excellent. There's always something available that can be tailored to your needs. And what would really boost this process is if the expectant parents also find a de-stressor they can do together to strengthen their own bond, as well as their pre-birth commitment to do what's best for their child.

One is led to ask, Why are so many people taking vaccines? Many mechanisms are implemented to get people to take vaccines such as laws requiring children to do so and mandates on government employees and military personnel.

Vaccines, by the way, are designed by virtue of the introduction of a live or dead virus into the body to induce the immune system to recognize the foreign invader and react accordingly, should a real infection occur. A small problem here, however—many viruses (with their own innate intelligence) have cultivated an enormous capacity for change (mutation) so that they can often "escape recognition" by the immune system over time. Therefore, vaccine usefulness, as I've seen in many of my patients who've received them, is questionable. Remember: A placebo is capable of eliciting a 30-percent rate of success (alone!). This may explain, in part, according to a survey done by *The American Journal of Nursing*, why **less than 40-percent of health care workers take vaccines despite urging by the Center for Disease Control (CDC).**

Too late for you to go back in time and change events, you say? Been blasted with round after round of these toxins and other poisons? You now have a means to help dispel these disease-causing agents. As you read on, the healthy choice you can take will become clearer and clearer. And, it is your choice.

Neuropathy and neurological and severe psychological problems, including depression, are very real problems related to heavy metal toxicity. Heavy metals such as mercury, interfere with the repair of DNA. This is according to many different studies. These metals also kill off friendly bacteria in our digestive tract; interfere with immune system function and endocrine gland function (including hormone secretion); neurotransmission (transmission of nerve impulses from the brain to the rest of the body which causes tremors, shaking, tingling, and numbness); debilitate the activities of enzymes (needed for all of the body's bio-reactions); deplete and destroy minerals such as zinc, magnesium, calcium, chromium; and negatively affect all cell membranes. They are implicated in many allergic reactions. In short, they can undo many of the holistic benefits we strive for by living right.

Before I leave the topic of vaccinations and heavy metal poisoning, I want to give you some findings of Dr. Hugh Fudenberg, a widely-quoted expert in medical and scientific literature and head of the Neuro Immuno Therapeutics Research Foundation. He reported some disturbing and startling findings at a vaccine conference in 1997—"If an individual has had 5 consecutive flu shots between 1970-1980 (my note: the years of his study), his/her chance of developing Alzheimer's Disease is *10 times greater* than if they had one or no shots (emphasis in italics are mine).

I've been a dentist for many years and am able to draw a correlation between people with poor dental health and poor general health. Dentistry is truly one of the most toxic professions imaginable. One dentist friend made an analogy that, "It is similar to repairing watches while someone is spitting on you." I've analyzed blood from dentists over the years and found indications of insanely high levels of mercury and other heavy metals. I've also noticed that people, in particular women, who have a large number of amalgam fillings, tend to have more difficulty with conception and the health of their children, in general. This is definitely an area begging for more research. Mercury poisoning can even produce symptoms often mis-diagnosed as Multiple Sclerosis (MS) and can mimic Lou Gehrig's disease.

When mercury from amalgam fillings leaches into our system—and, according to renowned experts, it most certainly does, despite claims by the medical authorities—and gets trapped by the blood-brain barrier, neurological disease can happen. People who work with or near mercury are at risk through actual and vapor contact. A growing number of European and Asian countries have outlawed the use of amalgams. There is an ever-widening movement to do this around the world. You can find dentists who will replace amalgam fillings with safer, less-toxic white fillings.

No surprise here—we don't see this movement against amalgam in the United States (fear of retribution); although, laws have been passed that require the disposal of scrap mercury in special bio-hazard toxic-waste containers when removed from the mouth. Yet, you still hear many dentists and the American Dental Association (ADA) state that amalgam is perfectly safe to place in a human mouth. The ADA, which refuses to ban amalgam—probably because they own the patent— warns dentists to know the potential hazards and symptoms of mercury exposure and not touch the substance. Recall that I stated earlier that the ADA, like the AMA, is not a governmental agency, but a trade union. Just follow the money, as is said.

You can't throw amalgam in the trash or bury it in a landfill, but you can put it into the mouth. Questionable, at the very least. For this reason alone, dentists should read this book from cover to cover and, at least, become aware of the risks of being in the profession. And, by the way, according to a very recent (2006) ruling by the FDA "panel of experts," it was ruled 13 to 7 that mercury-containing amalgams pose no health hazard. Doesn't that make you feel safer now? A search on the Internet can provide more information about this ruling.

Along with amalgams, perhaps one of the greatest threats to human health are root canals. I've done many of these, and have several of these, myself. Many degenerative diseases can originate from root-filled teeth. The most frequent are heart and joint diseases followed by brain and nervous system disorders, according to an investigation done in 1990 by Dr. Weston Price. This chilling investigation was based on 25 years of research conducted with a 60-man team.

Why this "focal infection?" When a tooth's root is dying from decay, disease, or other factors, it is cleaned out and filled, usually with what is called gutta-percha. While it looks great on the X-ray, the many microscopic lateral canals in the dentin of the root are never truly sealed. As a result, bacteria such as streptococcus, staphylococcus, and spirochetes set up a wonderful home in these areas, multiply, have families, and send their "children" out as new bacteria to play in the neighborhood or your inner organs. (Note: Ozone injected into teeth before completion of the root canal, has been shown to be successful at killing off these bacteria. Ozone used systemically, also helps kill organisms that manage to get into the body.)

Diseases such as arthritis and other crippling conditions, have cleared up remarkably with extractions of such teeth. As further proof, Dr. Price extracted root canal teeth, embedded these under the skin of a rabbit, and in two days, the rabbit developed the same kind of crippling arthritis as the patient. In ten days, it died—and this time, not from a pregnancy test! The rabbits always developed the same disease the patients had. If it was the heart, rabbits developed heart disease. If it was the kidney, the same pattern followed. Removal of the tooth almost always resolved the problem.

Going back to my training in Chinese medicine, it has been shown that each and every tooth occupies a vital place in the mouth through which meridians (described earlier), or energy channels, travel. Biological dentists recognize that bad dental work or poison-containing fillings set up an energy blockage at this level and short-circuit the entire energy loop of the associated organ system. Bioenergy measuring devices confirm this time and again. These meridians (described by Chinese, and probably Indian, sages) being affected, means that a problem in the tooth affects the corresponding organ. Experts in the field of biological dentistry have linked the deterioration to the development of even cancer, in time, believing that many cancers are related to "dental focus" factors. Conversely, disrupted energy in associated organs must be dealt with before the tooth or bone area around it can be successfully restored, if damaged. As an example, the upper and lower incisors (biting teeth) are related to the reproductive organs. When I have examined people with problems in these organs— i.e., cancer, reproductive difficulties, cysts, etc., I have almost always seen plaque build-up, gum problems, or loosening in these dental areas. Both must be cleared up for health to take place. This can be done bioenergetically; but, that is a subject for a whole different book.

I have seen remarkable improvements in patients' health after removal of toxic metal-containing fillings. I've seen even more remarkable levels of general systemic pain relief after I manually, through an impressive osteopathic adjustment technique I was taught and later expanded on, adjust the relation of the bite. This technique involves manipulation of not only the muscles, ligaments, and tendons, but of the bone sutures (connectors) in the mouth and temporomandibular joint region. I've seen headaches, ear problems, confusion, and even lower back pain disappear almost instantaneously. Incidentally, it was taught to me by a 90+-year-old doctor in a hospital in Tibet; and Tibetan medicine is said to have descended directly from Buddha and is called "Healing from the Source." A highly evolved doctor who practices this healing form is addressed as...Buddha.

People get caries (cavities) from poor diet, poor care, neglect, etc. Small cavities become bigger ones that sometime turn into root canals. Is it practical to extract all of these? Do you really want to look like some of the cartoon depictions of back-woods characters? What is the alternative? Keep your immune system high and kill off most of these circulating bugs in your system. Use good lifestyle management and, yes, don't sweat it—or, rather—Know Sweat! as part of the solution. Remember, we live in the real world; and, health is a matter of balance.

On a different note, if extraction becomes necessary, currently-used implants offer some degree of a bio-compatible solution. I am looking into the feasibility of using crystals implanted in the jaw bone, on top of which teeth can be placed. Can you imagine the energy of quartz in that area? You'd have the potential where the replacement might actually be as good, or better, bioenergetically, than the original!

Like everything else, metals work their way into fat tissues. Fat is one of the main toxic storage dumps of the body. By no means, though, are fat cells metabolic dead-weight cells. Fat releases fatty acids into the blood stream. Fat cells also generate proteins and hormones which are associated with a disease-causing and potentially dangerous process called "inflammation," a foundation for diseases such as cancer, heart disease, obesity, diabetes, and a host of other degenerative diseases. *Inflammatory cytokines* (destructive cell-signaling chemicals) such as TNF-alpha (tumor necrosis factor), IL-6 (interleukin-6), IL-1 b (interleukin-1 beta), IL-8 (interleukin-8) are associated with the all-too-common dangerous state of degeneration. This process, as noted before, promotes insulin resistance. Insulin levels rise as cells lose their ability to respond to insulin efficiently. As toxin-laden fat tissue increases, so does the risk of hyperglycemia (diabetes is not far behind) and a vast array of other diseases such as high blood pressure, and it elevates disease-causing blood lipids such as triglycerides and low-density lipoproteins (LDL), the dangerous ones.

Toxins quietly accumulate in fat tissue over years and remain there like ticking time-bombs. According to the Environmental Protection

Agency (EPA), fat biopsies contain not only mercury and poisonous metals, but also carcinogenic PCBs, styrene, dioxins, and other toxins. These impair the metabolism of fat tissue. This is also why when people do crash diets or yo-yo their weight up and down, the metabolism of their toxic fat tissues changes dramatically. This type of activity releases these substances into the body and toxifies the body. Because this dieting modality impairs the metabolism (it slows down because the act of dieting triggers an anti-starvation mechanism), once these individuals begin to eat more calories, especially fattening ones, the fat piles back on in larger quantities and becomes more difficult to lose, usually seen as those ugly-looking fat clusters located in the thighs and hips called cellulite. If you do not wish to greet the surgeon's cold steel scalpel, hit the far infrared sauna, capable of penetrating up to 1.75 inches into the body's tissues. It would help if people learn something quite simple about weight maintenance: Eat enough. Your metabolism needs enough calories to work properly, but of the right foods. Eliminate or minimize white foods—flour, rice, sugar, potatoes, dairy; and, you can easily maintain your proper weight. **Note: Body fat becomes water soluble at 110°F and can begin to get sweated out at this temperature.**

What about fluoride and chlorine placed into water supplies? In my opinion, these two are some of the major toxic culprits contributing to disease. While it is impossible to do a double-blind study to isolate and measure the effects of either—too many other variables—many studies suggest that while each have been cited to have some "beneficial" effects, i.e., fluoride in prevention of cavities and chlorine for water "sterilization," they are potent toxins to the body. Alternatives should be sought. It's important to remember that these two chemicals enter your body quite actively through your largest organ—the skin—when you shower or use a steam sauna. A typical shower allows six times more chlorine to enter the body than a day of drinking chlorinated water!

The National Academy of Sciences has determined that *fluorine*, a component of fluoride, slows DNA repair activity. Research at the Wisconsin Medical College and Harvard University has shown that chloroform-containing chlorine, the most common known as *trihalomethane*, is, indeed, a carcinogen. As time goes on, clean water may become more valuable than even oil. It stands the chance of being even more scarce and fought over than black crude. Rather than oil barons, we may have water barons. If wars can be fought over oil, they most probably will be fought over water.

In the September 13, 2006 online edition of the *Del Rio News-Herald* (Del Rio and Val Verde County, Texas), it was reported that the city council decided to remove fluoride from their water supply after a presentation by a retired biology professor, "...who characterized fluoride as a poison and showed the council numerous research references that link fluoride to higher rates of cancer and other health hazards." Why? "Basically for two reasons: fluoridated water cannot be shown to significantly reduce dental caries (tooth decay) and it has proved to be far more toxic than previously thought." I don't want to draw attention to particular products or their producers, but do notice some of the new fluoridated items that are being offered today—items that will impact current, and therefore, future generations.

What can we do? We clean up our act. We choose better foods (organic). We eliminate poor food choices. We filter our water for drinking and washing our bodies. And, we sweat deliberately. Regular sweat baths, along with lifestyle enhancement techniques, not only remove toxins but also prevent them from entrenching into fat tissues and other deep-tissue levels. Additionally, a hard-bristle brush usually found at health food stores, can be used to remove surface skin-cell accumulations. There are proper ways to use this type of dry-brush technique that not only smooth the skin, but stimulate the lymph system (especially behind the knees and neck). When you dry-brush, you always draw the brush in one direction and always in the direction of the heart, which follows the path of the lymphatic system. Don't use the brush on the more sensitive areas of the chest or face. If you do this prior to sweat therapy, you increase the effectiveness of the detoxifying process. This dry-brush technique, along with sweat therapy, can reduce or even melt away cellulite, depending on your diet.

A word of caution: The more toxic your body is, the more it will react to the initial act of being detoxified. Be patient. Pay attention to any symptoms that happen (headache, dizziness, sluggishness, skin blemishes, etc.). Initially, you may feel like you were hit with a two-ton brick in the face. You are also killing off viruses, bacteria, and parasites in your system which have caused you dis-ease. Your spirit and their spirit have formed some sort of, not-good-for-you, symbiotic relationship—a discordant harmony, if you will. Fascinating psycho/bio/spiritual/vibrational bonds formed by the parasite and host are well-documented in the field of parasitology. Most parasites even influence behavior patterns in the host through a very intricate and still poorly understood biochemical mechanism. The host actually begins to behave in accordance with a pattern beneficial to the survival and perpetuation of the parasite. This is well-documented in other species, as well. For example, snails normally live hidden, protected from most predators, in moist areas at ground level in the forest. Ingestion of a parasite makes them actively climb tall grasses which is a self-destructive pattern that goes against their nature. Birds then see them and easily pick them off the grasses, eat them, and defecate the eggs from the parasites to start the cycle all over again.

When you kill parasites—and no life, no matter how ugly-looking, wants to die—chemicals are released. This ends or reduces toxicity, and causes a biochemical and spiritual shift. If you studied microbiology and looked at some of these microorganisms under a microscope, you would run for the entrance to the sauna. You don't need special-effects people to create the next sci-fi horror film creatures. They're right there in front of (or in!) you.

Believe it or not, there is actually a grieving process that takes place. The crappy feeling people experience is caused by the dying parasitic masses releasing toxic crap as a farewell present to you for their (unhealthy for you) residing in your body. Remarkably, this can cause a sense of loss, grief, and sadness. Know that this is your body's initial response to releasing toxins that have been stored in fat and other tissues. Human nature generally resists change and loss—whatever the form. Thank God this is only temporary. It is a funeral, but shed no tears unless they are tears of relief (or release). These microorganisms demonstrate their tenacity for life through their future children or eggs left in your body, which must also be removed. Bless them all and let them go. As soon as the level of toxins reduce through sweat therapy (and any other adjunctive detoxifying process you use), your body will begin to re-balance itself. You'll soon feel better, sleep better, and actually seem to glow with healthier skin and overall health, in general. Dr. Hulda Clark (another person not popular with the allopathic medical community) has identified the presence of the eggs or organism, itself, of the liver fluke in 100-percent of all cancers she investigated. We can never rid the world of these, only our body—and only to some degree of success. Ultimately, we co-exist; but, there's no reason we cannot manage their levels and diminish their impact on us.

So, there you have it. **If you are even thinking of detoxification without a good sweat therapy program, don't do that—unless you are one of the rare individuals who should not sweat or needs to exercise certain cautions as described in various sections of this book.** As I said earlier, I've had the opportunity to study blood of over 50

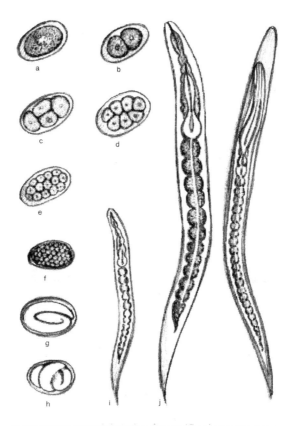

HOOKWORM IN ITS VARIOUS STAGES OF DEVELOPMENT

dentists with the result of seeing slides full of heavy metals, even when detox protocols like sweat therapy were added. **Anything you can do to reduce the toxic load on your body benefits you.**

As you've seen so far in this chapter, some very standard medical and dental practices can cause or trigger disease in your body. Sweat therapy and other healthful methods can, literally, help your body rid itself of most toxins and heavy metals introduced by virtue of trying to take care of your health! This is one primary reason people need the information in this book.

What About Stress?

Let's take a hypothetical situation—one that may not be so hypothetical for many, today. You've had a crazy time getting the kids off to school. Your head aches. Maybe you didn't sleep so well. You're worried about finances or something else. You get to the office and after your third cup of coffee or other preferred stimulant, hear the boss wants to see you right away. Just what you need. An alarm reaction starts in your body and the G.A.S. (general adaptation syndrome) kicks in. You just know this meeting is not going to be good. Your hypothalamus perceives an impending stressor. After a massive adrenaline release, the hypothalamus activates the sympathetic nervous system (fight-or-flight mode). The pituitary gland is on alert. The physiological effects on the body are now irreversible and have to run their course.

The stroke volume of your heart increases along with the rate and volume of blood flow. Blood vessels in the blood reservoirs (skin, kidneys, and most of the viscera) constrict. Skeletal muscle vessels dilate in preparation for fight or flight. Digestion slows to a minimum or stops. Adrenal glands kick into high gear. Epinephrine flows like a river, and your liver has stepped up (glycogenolysis) so you can have an instantaneous increase in blood sugar (hyperglycemia), which translates into rapid energy. Your brain waves are in the beta state—active, alert, rather than relaxed. You're mentally on the razor's edge. Your primitive reptilian brain counterpart has you standing inside your cave which is blocked by a fierce wooly mastodon that resembles your boss.

Your boss says your high-tech skills are needed to train a young, bright computer specialist for the next two weeks. It will be an intensive training. That's the good news. The bad news ("Oh, no, Mr. Bill!") is that your job has been out-sourced to Bangalore, India, and this talented trainee is your replacement. The boss says he understands your plight; but, this is a corporate situation and Human Resources may be able to help you adjust. Perhaps he apologizes. He wishes you good luck. You gaze out of the window as you think of something to say. The rush of adrenaline abates somewhat. Palpitations diminish a bit, but you are sweating. Oh, God—the needed trip—that cruise you had planned for years, the mortgage payment, your children's music lessons... After a short time, your mind and body progress to the second stage called *resistance*. Were these mechanisms to continue, you would experience wear-and-tear and suffer damage—possibly of a permanent nature. Cortisol (anti-inflammatory stress hormone) and aldosterone (increases sodium and water retention, contributing to blood volume) are secreted in excess.

You leave the office somewhat shell-shocked and your body progresses to the third stage characterized as *exhaustion*. The toxic by-products of stress hormones and neurotransmitters released into your system need to be broken down, transformed, and eliminated from your body. Your liver and kidneys need to be spared. What do you need to do? Yes. Know sweat! As soon as you get home, get into the tub or sauna and do some sweat therapy or do some exercise—maybe go for a long walk or, better, do both. You'll need a clear mind to contemplate how you will turn this event into an opportunity. Maybe this was the best thing that could have happened. Now you can start your own business. You can train others in the same way you are now expected to train your replacement. Only now, you can do it as your own enterprise. You may even start a chain. But you'll want to have as many as possible of the toxins that accumulated during this shift released from your body as quickly as you can. You want to make a plan for your future and take action with a clear head, strong body, and enough energy.

If your life has repetitive scenarios similar to this example, your health will deteriorate. We are not designed to live in constant stress.

The chemicals released, as described above, are for fight or flight only—not daily living. This is how burnout or exhaustion happens. It's what causes Chronic Fatigue Syndrome. And, it is something you want to avoid. If your job or life are high-stress ones (different from active where you love what you do), it is imperative that you do sweat therapy, in some form, at least three times a week to keep toxins from building up.

If you are unhappy or depressed, the very first thing to do is change your mood. Feeling discontent means you are probably not on the same "wavelength" as what is going on around you, right down to the vibrational frequencies of your body's water molecules. These opposing or out-of-balance frequencies manifest as antagonisms. You can make this your opportunity to elevate your level of vibrational energy. To paraphrase Einstein, No problem is ever solved at the same level it is created. You have to lift yourself higher in some manner.

Understand that emotions must be honored, so you don't want to disregard what you truly feel after an event that creates some kind of shock to your system. Just remember that motion changes emotion. As quickly as possible, release the shock and decide to take positive action that moves your forward. Otherwise, you cannot be healthy—plain and simple. Laughter has been shown to be an excellent starting point. Other things you can do to begin to de-stress yourself is to find and embrace a way to give thanks or feel appreciation for what you do have in your life, and do so on a consistent basis. Smile, laugh, give and receive hugs, and perform random acts of kindness to produce the kinds of chemical responses you want in your body. These acts take a circular path in the universe and find their way back to you. You reap what you sow—or in modern lingo, What goes around, comes around.

Some stress is necessary for life. You need to challenge bones, ligaments, and tendons with stress to keep them strong. You need to challenge emotions so that you gain insight. Challenge the mind so you learn more. There are healthy stressors just as there are friendly bacteria that help us stay balanced and well (they have their own good spirit too!). Healthy stress produces *endorphins* (endogenous morphine) and *enkephalins*, which are our internal immune-system boosters. The state of *no mind* achieved with qigong, yoga, or meditation can also produce this result. Much stress can be turned around to create mental, spiritual, and physical balance. Everything happens for a reason. You can decide to use every moment as an opportunity for personal growth, to waste nothing, and learn from everything that touches your life.

Also, avoid strong electromagnetic fields. **Try to minimize time spent with electromagnetic devices since this is one stressor which is virtually impossible to dissipate.** And, yes, negative people can also give you electromagnetic stress and disrupt your energy field if you let them. Try to avoid these types of people if they insist on remaining negative and pessimistic despite your sincere desire to help them. They can penetrate all of the four outer layers of your aura if you let them (see "*Shaolin Yoga: Qigong*").

As noted before, our energy field (aura), unseen by most but often seen by those open to seeing it, forms a subtle protective bioenergetic armor-like shield around us. This etheric-physical interface is what keeps the body in equilibrium with the external energies we are subjected to at any given time. Subtle changes in these such as electromagnetic pulses, lunar events, solar flares, eclipses, etc., produce affectations. Being bombarded by criss-crossing, piercing, penetrating and dangerous electromagnetic waves from man-made devices on a constant basis creates subtle changes in these natural bioenergy fields. Consider this next time a cell phone works inside a building or in an underground subway train—environments where you think you're free of electromagnetic pollution. The vibrational frequencies of these fields, our chakra system, and the artificially-imposed toxic energy of external man-made fields contrast with one another to co-exist at the same place and time. The body's protective energy (wei chi) breaks down. The natural orbits of electrons and protons in our cells' nuclei change. The bond angles of molecules such as water and its surface tension, are adversely affected.

The bioenergetic template gets set up for disease to penetrate every cell in our body. Contrary to what is said by "experts" in the industry, there is ample evidence to indicate that this electromagnetic disruption can and will, after a period of time and related to the strength of our bioelectric immune system, create gaps and disruptions not only generally, but more specifically, in the particular areas where they are directed, i.e., the temporal part of the brain as seen with cell phones. Each layer of the body's defensive electromagnetic field becomes pierced and altered until the damage that initially began at the bioenergy level, progresses to the atomic, then cellular, then tissue, then organ level. In the end, the bioenergetic stressor will create disease in this particular organ system.

One way to change this is to change the resonance of our own frequencies. The beneficial, disease-fighting frequency of a far infrared sauna seems to be one way. Flower remedies, homeopathic remedies, crystals (quartz, in particular), mind-body-spirit practices such as qigong and yoga are other means to accomplish this. Choosing to be happy, giving because you value your contribution and service to others, giving and receiving love, and true appreciation for all that blesses and graces your life raise your vibrational frequency to a more protective one. A true remedy is laughter—real belly laughs. Some aspects of life are serious and deserve to be dealt with as such. But really, most of what we treat as serious isn't as serious as we make it out to be. We'd do ourselves and others a true service if we learned to laugh more.

In summary, when we are stressed, the circulatory, nervous, endocrine, and immune systems are activated by toxic breakdown of stress by-products. This causes a psychological, physiological, and immunological response. This is why I always refer to mind-body-spirit detoxification as the best way. When the mind and spirit are poisoned by stress, emotional upset, and toxic emotions (the Seven Demons according to Chinese sages), the body suffers due to the metabolic degradation of these by-products. Furthermore, it was shown that negative thoughts actually have an effect on DNA. Constricted thoughts can constrict DNA, making it shorter, and switch off many of its codes. Telomeres, which pull apart DNA to create new DNA, become affected. This shortening eventually leads to early DNA death which has the potential to shorten other things, including our lives, since when we stop "dividing" and, thus, stop growing—like a plant or a cell, we stop living.

Stress is, in my opinion, a component of virtually every disease. Numerous studies have made the link between stress and its related psychological components and susceptibility to cancer. Traumatic changes in one's life, including loss of a loved one, divorce, or separation places one at a much greater risk for cancer. You can choose to treat stress with drugs, but if you can take a safer path, why not do so? Especially a path with no harmful side-effects. ***The Journal of the American Medical Association* (JAMA) estimates that over 125,000 Americans die each year from side-effects of FDA-approved drugs.** Some of these drugs are designed to "help" people cope with stress and its effects. Maybe you've noticed some of the newer commercials (2006) warn something like, "If you notice your depression worsening, contact your doctor. Also, people under the age of 18 have been known to experience suicidal effects from this drug."

Notice that I did not include a separate category for respiratory problems. Breathing is almost always taken for granted; yet, it is one of the most vital functions of the body. After you read, *"Shaolin Yoga: Qigong,"* you can begin to breathe like a monk—the right way! It is estimated that 92 million Americans—more than one out of three—suffer from one of the four most common chronic respiratory illnesses: Asthma, bronchitis, hay fever, and sinusitis. They are often characterized by congestion, coughing, and mucous secretion. Inasmuch as there is a definitive link between airborne pollutants and viral, bacterial, and fungal infections, internal (toxic) pollutants, along with parasites and their eggs, lodge into various regions of the respiratory system. These respiratory illnesses can be caused by deficiencies in the immune system and its protective elements, and can be a primary factor in weakening the immune system. Remember, *breath chi* is the vital life force in Chinese and Indian medicine. Stress makes a person's breathing choppy, shallow, and essentially ineffective in oxygen assimilation and toxin elimination. Breathing properly will help the energy flow in this area and prevent at least some of these poisons from settling in.

Deep breathing should be done while in a sauna, though practiced with caution. This helps bring the heat into the bronchi where it can begin to relieve inflammation and congestion of not only the upper, but lower respiratory tracts. Steam sauna use or inhalation is particularly effective since it moistens and relieves the irritability of mucous membranes. Heat also relieves spasmodic breathing as seen in croup or asthma, by virtue of loosening and dislodging much of the bacteria- and virus-harboring mucous. This allows heat to eliminate microorganisms that may well be the physical root of the problem to begin with. Finally, since the bronchial muscles relax, blood supply improves along with lymphatic and meridian-related chi flow, which helps expel a good deal of "debris."

Stress makes things worse and may actually be the precipitating factor in a respiratory condition such as asthma. Just ask someone who has a child with asthma. A growing body of research indicates that asthma attacks are triggered by stress, which leads to more stress being generated. As explained before, the body's immune system will break down and the cycle will continue. A detox program, along with some good old sweat therapy (are you beginning to "Know Sweat" yet?), may just be what the doctor ordered to boost the immune system.

Here's another one to think about: Cystic Fibrosis (CF). About 30,000 people in the U.S. have CF while twelve million Americans are carriers of the CF gene—an amazingly high, relative number. This condition is probably the ultimate manifestation of a mucous-related respiratory condition. Most common symptoms are salty-tasting skin, and lung, sinus, and gastrointestinal problems. In fact, it is the sweat test which is the most useful test for diagnosing CF, done by measuring the salt level in sweat. Because of the CF gene, sweat function is disrupted. This abnormal gene causes sweat to become extremely salty, causing the body to lose vast quantities of salt which, of course, upsets the mineral balance.

CF, as an inherited disease, affects mucous and sweat glands in both males and females. This disease impacts mostly the lungs, pancreas, liver, intestines, sinuses, and sex organs. Mucous found in the body is watery under normal conditions, and keeps the lining of many organs moist and prevents them from drying out or becoming infected. In CF, an abnormal gene causes mucous to become thick and sticky. The most common cause of death in CF is respiratory failure. Of notable concern, is the mucous build-up in the lungs. Airways become blocked. Stagnation takes place. Life-giving air chi is diminished. From this, a foundation for the growth of bacteria and other organisms is created. Health-threatening lung infections become more and more common. In time, the lungs become damaged. Stress makes this worse and the disease much harder to control by wreaking havoc on the already compromised immune system.

CF also affects the digestive system. The sticky mucous blocks pancreatic ducts, and function of digestive enzymes produced in the pancreas—so essential to break down and assimilate food we ingest—is hindered. We cannot absorb fats (blockage of lipase enzymes) or proteins (blockage of protease enzymes) through our intestines. As a result, we suffer not only from respiratory problems, but inefficient nutrient assimilation (malnourishment). If you read *"Shaolin Yoga: Qigong,"* you see that the respiratory/digestive system (lung/large intestine element) is part of the same system referred to as "the metal element," expanded in my second Health and Wellness Series book, *"Zen and the Way of the Sword."*

In the past, most CF sufferers did not live past their teens. Today, fortunately, we see greatly extended life spans. Once again, lifestyle management is the key to success—and survival. If someone you love has this condition, follow a sound nutritional protocol, keep faith, get them to do lots of qigong and/or yoga and—Know Sweat! Just go back and revisit the main enemies of mucous and infection: Heat and oxygen. Dr. Bill says, "It can be done!"

Allergies are no different. In fact, many of the body's respiratory problems may be linked, in some way, to allergies. Hay fever, or what is termed as allergic rhinitis, is just another form of this weakened immune system condition. The body releases antibodies called IgG, IgA, IgM, IgD, and IgE to combat the offending cause, called *antigen*. These often cause visible reactions in the body. Once again, a stressed out, weakened immune system overloaded by toxins, can bring you to this point. With the right fortification of your immune system and a sound detoxification program along with stress management, you may be able to skip the massive allergy medicine aisle at your pharmacy.

These intrinsic (internal) toxins are just as poisonous to your system as the environmental chemicals and metals described earlier. If you recall, also described earlier was how Native American Indians use sweat lodges for spiritual as well as physical cleansing. It's all a part of a whole. Your body is designed to respond with, and to, chemicals either absorbed or released internally. As in the stressful office example given several paragraphs back, when the body releases certain chemicals into its system, even though they are meant to help us function in emergencies, we still need to eliminate them once the emergency is over.

Sweat therapy, as part of a detox program, can stress the body in a methodical, controlled, and beneficial manner. A "sweat junkie"—which I hope you become once you finish this book, if not before—has physiological reserves to help us cope more readily with stress. Not really a bad addiction when you think about it. As I said, this reserve serves your cardiovascular, endocrine, and nervous systems. Medical treatment of anxiety and depression—conditions related to coping poorly with the stresses of life—focuses largely on the chemistry of neurotransmitters. I listed these earlier, but know that the actions of these chemicals are complex and quite different from one another. Once they perform their function, usually in milliseconds, their activity must be terminated or your body could literally be swimming in them. After a bit of chemical interaction takes place, the body needs to eliminate the by-products of these activities. No sweat? Yes, sweat!

Depression, as does its companion anxiety, has a strong biochemical basis and correlation. There is always some type of alteration in one or more of these neurotransmitters. In the general population, it's estimated by many experts in the field that there is a 15-percent prevalence of this experience at one time or another. People suffering from the stress of cancer can experience an increase in depression levels of 40- to 50-percent (*"Harrison's Principles of Internal Medicine"*). What is sad is that virtually every class of medication used to treat disease (anti-hypertensive drugs, anti-cholesterol drugs, anti-arrhythmic drugs) can actually trigger depression. This is because they elevate to toxic levels in your blood and the disease you are treating opens the door to other affectations or disease. Toxicity, once again! You can so very easily spare this overload on your major organs by simply sweating them out.

At the most basic level, depression is almost always caused by an incompatibility between our perception of what should be and what is. When these two do not jive, we feel powerless, helpless, and defenseless. There is conflict taking place. Hence, we have an illusion which helps create a delusion. Let's face it, with regard to events, "It is what it is." Sometimes, we cannot change situations—only find a way to come to terms and manage ourselves as best we can.

Sadly, some actually experience depression because of external physical factors. If you are not the "perfect" physical specimen, you may not become a fashion model. People who imagine they have some physical deformity or abnormality—termed Body Dysmorphic Syndrome—suffer a severe esteem-crushing, incapacitating belief that there is something wrong with their physical image that can never be made right. Nevertheless, in the infinite wisdom of the universe, you were probably given some outstanding artistic, spiritual, or intellectual qualities to offset this. These qualities are there! Focus on them rather than an obsessive pursuit of modeling contracts. Reassess your goals and do a reality check. Focus on your great qualities, enjoy these blessings, and rejoice.

And, I offer this: Always give. One of the surest ways to beat the blues and the peaks and valleys of anxiety attacks that may be interspersed within this potentially long, and sometimes very stressful cycle we call life—an upset that can ultimately affect your biochemistry and necessitate pharmacologic intervention for some—is to put others' needs before your own, i.e., the sick, poor, homeless, etc. Such action, in the form of true service, wakes you up and gives you a reality check. From personal experience, I can refer you to some of the neighborhoods where I took care of patients who lived in below-standard conditions, and still do, if not locked up in prison or confined to some other institution due to circumstances—some within their control and some not.

Sweat Therapy and Pain

Everyone has experienced a form of pain at one time or another. Pain reduces quality of life. I have been blessed with the privilege of treating over 10,000 patients in my practice, many who initially came to me with the chief complaint of pain. According to Dr. Edward S. Rachlin, who specializes in myofascial pain and fibromyalgia, chronic and recurrent muscle pain affects 10- to 20-percent of the U.S. population. Studies done in other Western countries indicate that chronic pain is the second most-common medical condition after upper-respiratory illness. It is responsible for physical deterioration (due to lack of exercise), sleep disorders, and other psychosocial and behavioral disturbances. Chronic pain affects not only the pain sufferer, but everyone in their circle. It is a $100+ billion-dollar-a-year business.

Numerous physiological and metabolic disturbances occur in patients who have chronic pain. There is decreased ATP, AMP, and ADP in the muscles (all energy-releasing factors) and lower muscle oxygenation. Neurotransmitters such as serotonin, enkephalin, norepinephrine, alpha-aminobutyric acid, as well as others that make you feel good, are decreased in patients with chronic pain. In short, pain will make you feel bad. Pain hurts! Dysfunction of the neurons (nerve tissues) of the hypothalamus (temperature regulatory center for the brain) is also experienced. Just as a hot bath relaxes, a good sweat and release of toxins will make you feel even better. And the more you do, the better you will feel.

This being said, pain does serve a useful purpose. It is a warning sign. Pain that lingers after an area heals, or generally after four to six weeks, becomes known as chronic pain. Chronic pain does not serve a useful purpose. It's interesting that while pain syndromes can be caused by dysfunction of glands or organs (i.e., diabetic neuropathy), chronic pain can actually lay the groundwork for major organ dysfunction. Although a review of all types of pain and their treatment is beyond what I give you in this book, I can give you some additional insight into it. When chronic pain exists, electrical impulses are sent to the reticular activating system (RAS) of the brain stem, and structures within it called the intralaminar nuclei. These are stimulated in the thalamus. This means there is a constant excitatory effect going on. Since these two areas are also essential for sound sleep, **this is why people in chronic pain never get a restful night's sleep**. The brain is never calm. The body doesn't get the opportunity it needs to repair and rejuvenate from illness or injury. This raises the stress levels during the day. It's a vicious cycle.

Stress leads to muscle tension and prolonged muscle tension leads to pain. It was demonstrated in controlled EEG studies (electroencephalogram, an instrument that measures brain waves) that an increase of alpha waves in stage 1 (indicating arousal), followed by an intrusion of alpha waves into delta waves, and decreased delta waves in stages 3 and 4, indicated non-restive sleep and higher arousals, awakenings, and decreased sleep time. A tense, fatigued mind leads to a tense, fatigued body. A build-up of chemical messengers needs to be neutralized by sleep. If this doesn't happen, it causes the body to be in a constant state of exhaustion and agitation.

According to Dr. Guyton, cerebrospinal fluid, blood, and urine of animals kept awake for several days, contain a substance or substances that cause sleep when injected into the ventricular (brain cerebrospinal fluid) system of other animals. An animal kept awake for several days has a build-up of muramyl peptide, a low-molecular-weight substance which accumulates in the body. When even minute amounts of this are injected into another animal, even a well-rested one, it falls asleep in only a few minutes and sleeps for hours. Therefore, prolonged wakefulness results in an accumulation of such factors. Sleep facilitates detoxification and neutralizes these factors and breaks them down.

Recent studies are pointing out the prevalence of ailments related to lack of sleep. High blood pressure, diabetes, and obesity are at the top of the list. People under 60 who sleep five or fewer hours a night are twice as likely to develop hypertension as those who sleep seven to eight hours a night, according to a 2006 study of about 5,000 men and women. A recent national sleep foundation survey found a link between little sleep and hormonal problems, along with diabetes, in women. The lack of sleep increases the risk for diabetes and increases the risk of heart attack by 45-percent, and risk for death from all causes by 15-percent.

Another research study indicated that women who reported getting five hours of sleep per night were nearly twice as likely to be obese as women who regularly slept about seven hours. Getting only four hours of sleep a night elevated the risk of obesity three times the normal rate. This is the outcome of a 2003 study done on 2,500 women under 49 years of age. I'm sure the statistics don't vary too much for men. All of these statistics are just too great to ignore.

Sweat therapy helps you get to sleep, stay asleep, and have a higher quality sleep. If prolonged sound sleep is not possible, which adversely impacts your pain-related disorder, sweat therapy can help reduce accumulation levels.

Sweat therapy done in the morning, however, has an immediate benefit. Personally, when I haven't had enough sleep, sweat therapy rejuvenates me to a higher-awakened level. This is one reason why a sauna or, at least, a hot shower first thing after doing my qigong and tai chi exercises, or after a long day can rejuvenate. You can either "clear the deck" upon rising, or by the time you are ready to go to bed, you'll rest better without the toxic chemical soup simmering in your body all day.

Many pain sufferers are afflicted by muscle spasms. This can be caused by localized areas of tender or toxic muscle knots called trigger points. Feel the tops of your shoulders after a stressful day and you know what I'm referring to. They can be found in all tissues of the body and often place pressure on nerves, which creates pain. These points contain copious amounts of metabolic and external toxins including lactic acid. The *Bi-digital O-ring Test,* widely used by Dr. Yoshiaki Omura, demonstrates the presence of large amounts of heavy metals, especially mercury, in these trigger points. This was confirmed by urine analysis. You may literally be carrying the weight of the (toxic) world on your shoulders without realizing it.

An extreme case of this generalized pain is called *fibromyalgia* (more about this condition in Chapter 12). Blood flow and flow of what Eastern sages called chi or prana—what we normally call "life energy," are greatly diminished in the areas where pain occurs. There is a bioenergetic blockage going on. A reflex signal going to the spinal cord is activated, and by way of reflex feedback, muscle contraction results—a protective mechanism. The end-product is stagnation, toxicity, and pain. There are many different treatments for pain (mainstream and non-mainstream) ranging from nutrition, hypnotherapy, chiropractic, massage, biofeedback, acupuncture, energy medicine, hydrotherapy, injections, and even surgery—to name a few.

Sweat therapy should be part of every pain and stress management protocol used. The heat and circulatory effects do wonders in drawing out the lactic acid which relieves muscle cramps. The heat, as mentioned before, also activates the body's scavenging immune system cells and helps remove toxic waste products lodged in painful arthritic joints and other areas of the body. Blood vessels become dilated and greater circulation and higher levels of rejuvenating oxygen reach the injured areas. It also raises the level of the body's intrinsic (internal) natural anti-inflammatory—cortisone.

A unique situation experienced monthly by many women is menstrual pain. I don't want my fellow cro magnon men to feel slighted at this point. I will cover an array of pain syndromes for everyone, including those more applicable to men, in an upcoming book on pain management.

Humans were created with a unique, specialized organ system designed to ensure perpetuity of homosapiens on Earth—that is, if we cease to damage the planet to such a point that we destroy ourselves. The one we're addressing now is the female reproductive tract. Normal reproductive function depends on integrated action of the central nervous system, endocrine glands, and reproductive organs. In normal ovulation, somatic symptoms during the first few days prior to menses (the period) can present women with edema (water retention), breast engorgement, and lower abdominal pain—sometimes insignificant, and sometimes bad enough to be disabling. We have (experts believe) put man on the moon, but still cannot effectively treat, much less understand, PMS syndrome. Heat therapy, in some form, provides women relief from menstrual pain and has done so over the centuries. When asked if sweat therapy is good for menstrual cramps, I can only give you my feelings based on limited scientific data.

By the way, there are very interesting menstruation-related ramifications to therapeutic bathing or sweat ceremonies in different cultures. The mikvah, or ritual cleansing bath used in Judaism for cleansing the body, is done after menstruation and childbirth. The ghusl, which signifies ablution via a purity rite done after menstrual bleeding, intercourse, the first acceptance of creed or semen emission (in Islamic tradition), refers to cleansing and purifying after menstruation. I have not been able to find any significant consensus on recommendations for pain-relieving cleansing during the menses. We do know two things: Heat increases blood flow and submersion in cool to cold water temporarily slows or halts blood flow.

There's been a long-standing practice of using heat to relieve menstrual cramps whether by heating pad, the hot-water bottle of yesteryear, or taking a warm bath. Since heat creates molecular expansion and primes the body to detoxify itself, the relief is more than likely caused by loosening congestion in the female reproductive system. The lining that built up during the month in preparation to receive a fertilized egg, needs to be removed from the body, which is the partial purpose of menstruation. This, combined with the simple act of relaxing the body rather than tensing in response to painful cramps, may have all to do with why this works. With proper hygienic preparation, there's no reason not to do a sauna or sweat bath while a woman is menstruating. Women need to be aware that flow will probably temporarily increase during and just after sweat therapy. We're talking about women with normal flow patterns, not those with abnormal conditions that are more like hemorrhaging. Women who have such conditions will benefit by doing sweat therapy during the interval between menses, until the condition is resolved.

Use of infrared sauna has been shown to diminish lower back pain, as well as referred pain, and relief of cramps associated with the menstrual cycle. At the other end of the time spectrum, we should note that "hot flashes" during menopause, a sign that the hormonal system is trying to re-balance itself, can be helped with the beneficial effects of heat therapy on the endocrine and immune systems.

Massage often works well in conjunction with sweat therapy in the treatment of any pain syndrome. I recommend a protocol of 15-20 minutes of sweat therapy, followed by massage or any other form of body work, concluded by one or two 15-20 minute sweat therapy sessions. You want to open up sweat glands and pre-warm skin so that when the therapeutic effect of the massage readily releases toxins and poisons from muscle and fat tissues by mechanical stimulation, the sweat glands are primed to release massive amounts of disease-causing chemicals from the body.

There is still debate over whether heat or cold is beneficial for pain conditions. Both heat and cold are commonly used to reduce painful muscle spasms secondary to skeletal or neurological problems. The firing of neurons, indicating heightened muscle or organ activity as found in a painful condition, is diminished by raising the body's temperature only 2°F! It completely abates at an elevation of 7°-8°F. Heating of the skin, localized or generalized, removal of toxins, and a mechanism of anti-inflammatory response is achieved.

Based on my clinical observations, cold seems to work well in certain conditions, perhaps by its counter-irritant nature. Ethyl-chloride spray, commonly used to treat these types of body knots, has a similar effect. In clinical practice, I have broken up pain-referring trigger points with injections, acupuncture, and other high-tech energy-emitting gizmos to relieve pain. A great book on this topic exists, entitled, *"Myofascial Pain and Dysfunction: The Trigger Point Manual,"* coauthored by the late, great, grand lady of medicine, Dr. Janet Travell. She was also John F. Kennedy's private doctor (we can only imagine what information she had to keep to herself). A very important note to consider is this: When these knots are broken up, where do the toxins go? Some are readily eliminated and some are not, so they go right back into the system unless they are eliminated, traveling back to the energetically depleted and blocked areas creating new trigger points all over again. You can change this pattern by changing the way the body moves via *Feldenkrais* or *Alexander* movement technique, qigong, yoga, tai chi, or other body-movement forms. You can detoxify and send pain-related toxins and other chemical by-products right out of the body with—sweat therapy, of course!

Most people with chronic pain become so distraught with their condition, they withdraw and become pain-focused, inactive, fatigued, and eventually socially outcast and depressed as a result. No one wants to hear someone complain incessantly when you ask them how they are doing. As a rule, we prefer to be around people who exude powerful, positive energy. Sweat therapy raises the level of endorphins and helps a person feel better. Mood-enhancing neurotransmitters found abundantly in cerebrospinal fluid, by virtue of increased blood supply to the brain, are produced in even higher quantities since blood supply to the choroid plexus—the interface area between the circulatory system and ventricles (hollow CSF-producing and containing areas of the brain)—is increased in our highly-touted therapy. Greater blood flow means greater metabolism. This translates into higher production levels of this fluid that is rich in chemical messengers. The brain produces 500cc of this a day, but can only house 150cc. The excess gets sent out to positively influence the rest of the body by mechanisms I explain in more detail in my upcoming book, "Qigong Prescription," a book that is designed to make you feel good! This is a good first-step in breaking the cycle. Many routinely run to doctors for pain and depression medications, when they should also give consideration to running for the saunas and engaging in other sweat-producing activities. But this recommendation is not likely to be made via standard health care. Unfortunate, really.

Sweat Therapy and Addictions

Having grown up at the tail-end—or maybe it's the "never ends, just changes substances"—of the free rockin', lovin', druggin' culture, I have seen the ravages of many types of addictions. Many of my high school friends ended up having "bad trips." Some overdosed. Others... Well, they're just not who they used to be. To see such sensitive, loving but hurting souls devoured by this soul- and spirit-destroying demon is heartbreaking. This left an indelible imprint on me and I have always kept a part of my professional "practice" dedicated to this affliction. I never offer judgment, only help when they need it.

Thus, during the early 1990s, I started the first acupuncture and alternative medicine-based drug and alcohol rehabilitation program in a private New York medical center. I also established protocols and trained the counselors and social workers for Eric Clapton's legendary substance abuse program called *"Crossroads"* at Antigua, British West Indies. Eric Clapton is one of my heroes since, being a professional musician as I indicated before, I played bass guitar, among other instruments, in various bands. I grew up on Clapton's music. This was my chance to pay him tribute in a different way.

What is addiction? It is a chronic disorder which involves biological, biopharmacologic, and probably to some degree, genetic factors. Basically, it is a physical, psychological, spiritual dependency that negatively impacts one's life. We repeatedly use a substance or go back to a behavior, despite clear evidence of harm from it. It appears that whatever demon we have chosen, takes over our mind, body, and spirit. Often, we believe our power to resist it has been taken away. In reality, nothing can be farther from the truth. We always have a choice. Nevertheless, making the right choice can sometimes be painful in the short-term.

Although the major addictive substances cited over and over include drugs, alcohol, cigarettes, gambling, sex, reckless behavior, and over-eating, I can assure you that the varieties I have seen are only limited by the scope of the, sometimes bizarre, imagination. They all have a common thread in that the addictive substance becomes the necessary ingredient—a vital component of the body's own chemistry. It gets intertwined not only into the physical and mental component since "addictive personalities" demonstrate flaws in the brain's decision-making center, but also, in my observations, into the actual spirit, soul, or essence of the person. These substances fuse with the vibrational energy of a person's DNA.

One does not wake up one day and say, "Today, I will begin my addiction." Instead, it usually and innocuously, begins with a single drink, a single hit of a drug. Perhaps, maybe taking a prescribed drug that your doctor gave to you and, unfortunately, is how many addictions begin. No drug is ever really safe. A single thought can lead to a single act.

It can be said that everyone is addicted to something or other. I don't think there is an exception. It could be as benign as chocolate! The poison of choice, if you will, can be mild, hardly exacting a toll on our functional reality or in the extreme, can debilitate both the self and those around the individual. Quite often, it takes pain, real pain, to come to grips with this and make the necessary change. Remember that we are guided by two principles: Attainment of pleasure and avoidance of pain. Most of the time, the body, with its amazing resilience and infinite wisdom, can bounce back even from its shell-shocked state.

For those who don't believe in the organizing force of the universe, mentioned before, they quite often find IT in their most anguished moments of pain, when addiction threatens to take away everything that is dear, including life. Those who have not given too much thought to God or this universal force, quickly begin to embrace such thought...and, right at about this point in time. I have helped detox many individuals and find that from what I have witnessed, the common threads are the "angels," the spiritual beings who assist when a person sincerely, from the heart, makes a commitment—down to the molecular composition of the DNA's consciousness. Without including the cooperation of the spirit, one can be lost. This is at the core to get the demonic "monkey" off their back. All the rest, such as Twelve Steps, therapy, acupuncture, etc., are great adjunctive therapies, but remain simply adjuncts compared to the connection and commitment described here.

Having served as the Director of Anesthesiology and Pain Management in several programs at major New York City teaching hospitals, I've given my share of general anesthesia and intravenous sedation to many patients. This often induced analgesia; but for some was an unbelievable sense of euphoria—a real high. I could see how many weak individuals could get to like this sensation. Some even tried to return for benign dental procedures just to get high. One guy, right after I began to give him his I.V. sedation "cocktail," lit up with a weird smile and said, "Oh, man, this is great. I feel like I'm right back in Vietnam. Give me some more." Extreme care must be practiced by health care providers so as to not cause or exacerbate the problem.

Another very dear friend's son whom I've been treating since he was 3 and is now 25 years old, began a slow decline into hell and potential suicide. This journey began innocently enough after an oral surgeon prescribed Percocet, which he became addicted to after wisdom teeth extraction. At the time of this writing, his life just recently straightened out after going through the New York Center for Detox's proto-col. For all of those we can save, unfortunately, there are others a doc-tor sometimes is powerless to help.

The natural stimulants in the brain (catecholamines) and relaxants (endorphins) are often lacking in those with addictions. Neurotransmitters, mentioned before, may be lacking, as well. Thus, these substances provide an artificial type of stimulation which make you feel good. Decision-making skills become diminished—"What the hell, another drink won't hurt. My house is only a five-minute drive away." In a part of the brain called the ventromedial prefrontal cortex, your brain function becomes impaired and you're on your way—and maybe not to your own home, but into a tree or an on-coming car. One of my favorite television programs was "Twilight Zone." Each episode, Rod Serling would open with the word *Somewhere*—which is where someone under the influence will wind up, and perhaps not where they want to be—like intensive care or the grave.

A growing number of experts believe that there is a strong correlation between an allergy and becoming addicted to a substance. For exam-ple, we can become addicted to certain foods and continue to eat them in order to diminish the withdrawal symptoms, which would, of course, make us feel "bad." Thus, the allergy-addiction syndrome. Many experts also postulate that lack of a gene that breaks down alco-hol, may very well be the decisive factor in the high rate of alcohol addictions in Native Americans. Since allergies are an immune system problem, remember what your own "Dr. Detox" (as more and more people are beginning to address me as) has said about the relationship between allergies and poor immune response.

I have used complex vibrational-frequency tools to test food allergies such as Reinhold Voll's *Vegatest*, which is a machine that measures the bioelectrical energies traveling through the body's meridian system, with potential to indicate altered frequencies as an alert mechanism of impending disease. A phenomenal new machine that tests the body's vibrational frequencies in a whole new way is the EPFX (Scio). I'll be writing a book on it in the near future. To whet your appetite—think *"Star Trek."* I can also recommend a very easy, low-tech and extremely effective tool to test your allergy response. This is called the *Barnes Pulse Test.* Within half-an-hour to an hour of consuming a food, if your pulse starts to race by approximately 20-percent or more, you are allergic to that food. Plain and simple. You can isolate your favorite foods one-by-one and become very surprised at the results.

Sugar is one of these "foods." A sugar addiction may actually be the body's attempt to replenish serotonin levels in the body. Serotonin is a naturally-produced, calming, pain-killing chemical secreted in response to carbohydrate and sugar production. Unfortunately, persons who crave high amounts of sugar—usually originated through, of course, permission to children to indulge in this substance by parents who don't know any better (and some who do)—often have the potential to become addicted to alcohol as their opiate of choice later on. Alcohol not only has a high sugar content, but dulls the senses, providing temporary and potentially dangerous escape from feeling bad—a double whammy. Supportive of this is that many recovering alcoholics turn to sweets once they're no longer drinking. Their bodies crave the sugar high.

Ethanol, the component of drinking alcohol, is a central nervous system (CNS) depressant which decreases the activity of neurons. Many tout a glass of wine for its health benefits (i.e., resveratrol—an antioxidant in the Mediterranean diet). The alcoholic goes far beyond this. Tolerance develops and more and more of the "drug" is needed to satisfy the body's rapidly adapting hepatic defense mechanisms. Then, we see the full-blown syndrome. It may surprise you to know that most alcoholics are not people who live on the street. Only 5-percent of alcoholics do so.

Each substance has its peculiar pharmacology. While cocaine, processed from the leaves of the coca plant (erythroxylon coca) prevents the re-uptake of substances called biogenic amines, opiates work by a different mechanism (the euphoria from cocaine blocks dopamine re-uptake and also influences norepinephrine and serotonin). Opiates are in the group which consists of heroin, morphine, codeine, and derivatives. They bind to opioid receptors in the body and produce euphoria, sedation, and ultimately psychological and physical dependence. Tolerance, dependence, and addiction take place as more and more of the drug becomes necessary. The natural "fits" for the grooves of these receptors are, of course, the body's own naturally-occurring opiods such as enkephalins, endorphins, dynorphins, and others. Mind-body-spirit exercises and heat therapy naturally increases these endogenous chemicals in your body. You can create your own, natural high with no harmful short- or long-term negative side-effects.

What about smoking? Although I have a moderately good success rate for getting people to stop, don't think this is a mild addiction. Cigarette smoking is the principal cause of preventable disease, disability, and premature death in the U.S. "Scientists" (who should read the oath at the beginning of this book) carefully test and blend ingredients to maximize their effect on the body's receptors. More than 4,000 substances that are antigenic, cytotoxic, mutogenic, and carcinogenic, have been identified in cigarette smoke. It is one of the toughest addictions to break. I know. I used to smoke.

Virtually all of these addictions deplete the body's vitamins, minerals, and nutritional uptake mechanisms. You are literally starving yourself to death with the "chosen" monkey. And one more thing: Where do you think a great part of the metabolites of the addictive substances go after they interact with the body? Right into the fat tissues where they are stored, often as crystals and sludge in and between the adipose tissue, and can be found as many as 10 to even 40 years later. To a lesser degree, they can also be found in other connective tissue.

Along with counseling, a nutritionally-guided sweat therapy regimen is a must if you are to remove the toxic residue of addictions. Saying that sweat therapy will help kick the habit, so-to-speak, is an oversimplification. However, with all the other guidelines I've given (and will continue to give in up-coming books until this becomes a consciousness-changing alarm clock in people's minds), **some form of sweat therapy should be an essential cornerstone to free an individual from addiction. Any drug rehabilitation program not implementing this is missing out on a vital tool.** Remember everything we spoke about before: Sweat therapy strengthens the immune system. Mental, physical, and spiritual endurance and resistence to weakness is overcome. It detoxifies not only drugs, but virtually everything else out of the body and the body's receptors. It, plainly, makes you feel good—which is what the addicted person is looking for to begin with. Do it in a spiritual setting, such as Native Americans do, and you will get an incredibly amazing benefit. An addicted person's prayers may very well come true: Freedom from addiction and restoration of whole-self balance.

Many former addicts, including LSD users, re-live the original experience as the sweat therapy flushes the toxins out of their storage tissues and back into the circulation. This uncomfortable, short-lived experience is beneficial and is a milestone on the road to healing and wellness. Supplementation with Vitamin C, B-complex, magnesium, calcium, potassium, zinc, Bach Flower and homeopathic remedies, Chinese herbal teas, and chromium have shown great success when included in the detox treatment. Acupuncture therapies along with Chinese and ayurvedic liver cleansing herbs are also quite helpful.

The same can be said for the "detox" of a person whose had chemotherapy (another poison) in the past for treatment of cancer. At some point during their detox treatment, these patients begin to "taste" the chemotherapy agent as it diffuses out of their (toxic) storage tissues on its way to being expelled.

Don't forget, however, that once you remove the substance which (dangerously) makes you feel good, you must substitute something else to actuate the body's feel-good chemicals naturally. The euphoria once obtained through the substance, must be replaced by something that is, hopefully, naturally as good or better. Such euphoria registers in the nucleus accumbens—the "pleasure" area of the brain—and leads to the release of GABA (gamma-aminobutyric acid—a neurotransmitter associated with feeling good).

A little factoid for you: According to recent research, the right kind of music can stimulate this center and release many of the feel-good chemicals. Music therapy is a great natural and highly beneficial therapy. Many detox programs implement running. I strongly advocate yoga, qigong, or other spirit-based martial arts. When these are done while listening to the right chakra-harmonizing music, the benefit can be extraordinary. I'm sure if monks had access to recorded music in the old days, they would have taken advantage of it. Perhaps they had someone chant or play a musical instrument while they practiced. Select something that allows you to substitute good for bad.

Sound is vibrational frequency—audible light waves. Therefore, it's not a stretch to understand why sound is a form of vibrational frequency medicine, even if in the range the human ear can't hear.

Pleasingly organized sound—music—has been known for its healing effects for millennia. Oliver Wendell Holmes, Sr., American physician and poet (1809-1894) said, "Take a music bath once or twice a week for a few seasons, and you will find that it is to the soul what the water-bath is to the body."

An RN affiliated with Texas A&M University researched sound and, in particular, music, tracing its deliberate use at death, back to around 900AD (this is as far back as this specific recorded history was available to her). What she found was there are two "instruments"—and only these two—that should be used to soothe a person's release from this life to the next: The human voice and the harp. She also found the choice of sounds or notes and how they are organized musically significant, as well. Her motivation for this research was to find a means to help those in transition do so with dignity and as much serenity as possible. Music wasn't the only means she arrived at, but she found it is, indeed, important.

Resonating water molecules with the right frequency-range sound can negate negative frequencies associated with chemical imbalances. Experience of any type of sound triggers a tissue response to the positive or negative aspect. As the waves resonate through the body, crystalline structures of the tissues transform these vibrations into bioenergetically pulsing currents. These currents react with (or respond to) the energy fields in the meridians and organ systems. When sound is favorable, energy becomes regulated. If you think what you just read is nonsense, think about how your body and mind respond to a babbling brook as opposed to a jack-hammer.

The vast majority of the body is composed of water. In his book, *"The Secret Life of Water,"* amongst his other impressive works, Dr. Masaru Emoto stated and demonstrated that water has the quality of retaining vibrational frequencies (and, hence, emotions) of not only thought and word, but of vibrationally organized healing sounds called music. It's possible to positively affect the spirit of the body by listening to beneficial music. Music penetrates our psyche—one reason you may either hum or sing something you heard hours before, but it seems to be stuck in your mind. Dr. Emoto showed repeatedly, through meticulously-taken photographs of frozen water crystals at the precise moment when the phase is shifting from liquid to ice, the crystalline images that form when water was subjected to intense negative thoughts and words such as, "I hate you," as compared to more harmonious and beneficial thoughts and words of "Thanks" and "Love."

This same harmonious vibrational frequency of beneficial music (and thoughts and words) resonates the water and, hence, cells of our bodies to align us with higher, more beneficial frequencies—what some consider the universal consciousness' frequency of unconditional love. Dr. Emoto has done amazing research on sounds that heal joint injuries, depression, and other conditions. Lay people may not understand the principles, but the time-tested longevity of a spiritual and cellular-resonating piece, *"Amazing Grace"* by John Newton or *"Ave Maria"* by Schubert, have endured as songs loved by many who are moved not just by the lyrics, but by the musical compositions, themselves.

Withdrawal is a critical time. Dysphoria, the opposite of euphoria, will occur as the critical part of the nucleus accumbens' activity declines. This leads to anxiety, depression, and craving. Depending on the drug's elimination half-life (the amount of time necessary for the drug or agent to be reduced to half of its original level), this elimination process could be rapid or slow. Many drugs, recreational as well as prescription, can cause rebound effects which are a significant return to the original symptoms in absence of the original cause. This can cause depression. And remember, not only are the residues found in fat tissue where it's most concentrated, but can be found in all tissues. With the right mind-body-spirit cooperation, this will pass. Dr. Bill says, "Sweat it out!" As the Holmes quote suggests, supplement this with a pleasing music bath—not just to manage addictions, but stress, as well.

One more thing—and this, again, is my own opinion and based on my observations—don't forget about the angelic beings, which I touched on before. They touch my life every minute of every day. You may not be aware of it, but they touch yours, as well. These beings carry the medicine of divine creation. This *medicine*, if you open to it, will touch your soul and heal your spirit. This is much stronger than anything which can be synthesized in a laboratory. Carry their medicine in your medicine bag and let these spiritual beings who have a human experience into your life. You'll know who they are when you meet them. Hopefully, the world of healing will continue to attract more and more of these. They are your spirit guides, guided by love and compassion—your way out of the hell.

What Is the Ion Effect?

For at least 50 years, scientists have studied the effect of ions on our health and it's an area that deserves dedicated research. Some people use ion air-filtering machines in their homes. High amounts of negative ions in the air we breathe are very beneficial. An example of this is how we feel in the mountains after a thunderstorm has ionized and purified the air. Or when we are near a waterfall or any rushing waters, in the shower, or near an indoor or outdoor fountain.

Ions are electrically-charged molecules. The charge may be positive or negative. A molecule can gain or lose charge, thereby becoming its opposite in the process. In oxygen therapies such as ozone therapy, oxygen loses an electron then searches for another molecule. When it finds it, that molecule becomes negatively charged. In the process, a large degree of oxygen is released. This creates a vast aerobic environment and unprecedented healing within the body. Pioneering treatment for life-threatening diseases such as cancer or AIDS is based upon this in the field of oxygenation therapies.

Conversely, a high ratio of positive ions are detrimental to our health. An over-abundance of positive ions in the air resulting from closed-up indoor living, poor air quality, and air-conditioning can be harmful not only to our health (less fresh air circulation, reduced air quality), but also promotes agitation and irritability.

Negative ion therapy has been used in Europe and Russia for many years as an integral part of disease-treatment protocols. Negative ion generators not only help us feel better, but balance our bodies bioelectrically. This can prevent disease from forming at the most basic level. Disease first starts at the vibrational (DNA) or molecular level, proceeds to the cells, then tissues, then organs, then throughout the body. Sweat therapy that is induced by steam from water hitting heated rocks, produces abundant negative ions. Far infrared sauna therapy also creates this effect.

This chapter has been filled with a lot of medical terminology and explanation, though I promise I held back some—well, a great deal, actually. The purpose of this book is to invite you to open your mind to additional therapies, if you haven't already. There are more similarly informative books coming!

I think it's clear now that many methods exist to detoxify the body and why sweat therapy is an important part of any detox program. You can do it at home, so expense is not a problem. A bathtub and baking soda will do the trick at the most basic level. As I mentioned, my intention is not to frighten you with all that can happen when the body experiences the affects of toxic accumulations, but to give you enough information so that you can either consciously participate in proper health maintenance or in the restoration of healthy balance if you are either generally unwell, seriously ill, or somewhere in-between. My passion and purpose in life is to share every healthful and beneficial modality I can to help members of my human family heal and stay well.

"No one has ever drowned in sweat."   — Lou Holtz

SWEAT CONDITIONS:
Conditions Benefitted by Sweat Therapy

After the lengthy discussion you've read to this point,
this is the shortest chapter in the book.

Which conditions are benefitted by some form of sweat therapy?

With very rare exceptions—*all of them!*

(Apologies to the non-believers. I just couldn't find too many
conditions that wouldn't be helped by this.)

"If I had known I would live so long,
I would have taken better care of my body."
George Burns (somewhere in his 90s)

SWEATING: THE CHOICES

Methods to produce hyperthermia and sweat therapy induction, range from the ridiculously simple poor man's technique to high-tech, complex machinery. The end-product is always a rise in body temperature (fever) and sweat production. By far, sauna therapy seems to be the most popular, with saunas structured out of many materials such as cider and poplar. Steam baths seem to be equally popular.

At the other end of the spectrum, you can choose therapies that seem to go a bit into the extreme such as hallucinogenic shamanic ceremonies. But these are extraordinary and not easily fitted in between morning coffee and work. Unless you seek to expand your consciousness somewhere in the Amazon, this should not be your first choice. Ayurvedic (Indian) techniques, wrapping yourself in blankets with warm water bottles, or immersion into a hot-water bath are also options. If you live in an area where someone reputable holds sweat lodge ceremonies, that's something you can do on some consistent basis; but, you still want the option of getting a really good sweat going more often than that (three to four times per week).

Therapeutic baths (in a tank) are sometimes referred to with names like Schlenz, Sitz, Kneipp, and Hubba. Although some of these people, like Sitz in particular, are remembered for the bath named after them, one notable figure who stands out is Dr. Sebastian Kneipp (1821-1897). He was a Bavarian priest and a founding father of the naturopathic movement. His system, called the "Kneipp cure," is still in effect. Many sick persons were, and are still, returned to health via his five important tenets. These are

1. Hydrotherapy (hot/cold alternating-temperature baths)
2. Herbalizing
3. Exercise
4. Proper nutrition and, of course
5. Spirituality

For those of you unfamiliar with these particular baths, they involve immersing the body and sometimes just specific parts of the body, as in the case of prostate or uterine dysfunctions, and adding hot water into a bath that already contains lukewarm water. Increments of heated water are added until the tolerance point is reached and the therapeutic result is achieved. Sometimes warm drinks are taken during the course of one of these baths to speed up the sweating process. Because water prevents evaporation and cooling, a person tends to sweat profusely after leaving the bath. This is a time where you either need to remain unclothed or wear a terrycloth robe until the sweating subsides. Otherwise, you'll change clothes several times. It is, in fact, best if once you get out of the bath, you rest until the sweating stops, then enjoy a therapeutic nap or full sleep afterwards. In high-tech settings such as hospitals, diathermy—use of radio-frequency electromagnetic energy directed to the body, is yet another technique that causes a temperature rise and some sweating.

Mentioned in Chapter 5, radiant heating devices using infrared energy are a recent development and becoming popular in the United

States for the treatment of cancers, detoxification, and rehabilitation. As described earlier, a type of infrared therapy called Far Infrared Wavelengths (FIR) has begun to be utilized more widely in the last few years. Just do an Internet search for far infrared therapy and you'll see a rather big business. These wavelengths occur just above the visible red light in the electromagnetic spectrum (see diagram). FIR are reported to produce biologically beneficial vibrational effects on the body.

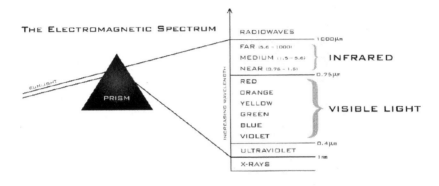

ILLUSTRATION OF FAR INFRARED WAVES WITHIN THE ELECTROMAGNETIC SPECTRUM,
COURTESY OF HIGH TECH HEALTH, INC.

Dr. Toshiko Yamazaki has done extensive research on uses of far infrared and provides some great insight into its mechanisms. In her book, *"The Science of Far Infrared Therapies,"* she indicates that the benefit of FIR in treating disease is that it removes toxins which are, of course, at the core of many health problems. These toxins are stored in our bodies since we are "bio-accumulators." According to her, toxic gasses such as sulphur dioxide, carbon dioxide, and toxic substances such as lead, mercury, or chlorine come into contact with large water molecules and are encapsulated by the clusters of water. In the areas of these toxic accumulations, blood circulation is blocked and cellular energy is impaired. However, upon application of 7-14 micron FIR waves to these, the water starts to vibrate. The vibration reduces the ionic bands of the atoms which hold together the mole-cules of water. With this breakdown of the water, encapsulated gasses and toxic materials are liberated and can more easily be eliminated. The effect of the particular wavelength of the FIR in countering and refracting the vibrational frequencies of disease entities is an exciting area that I'm sure will be studied more in-depth in the near future.

In contrast, short wavelength waves such as X-rays and gamma and alpha waves can damage the body. **FIR wavelengths are at the safe end of the wavelength spectrum and can penetrate the body up to one-and-three-fourths inches.** In actuality, the electromagnetic spectrum is divided into three segments based on micron wavelength measurements. Near infrared is approximately .076 to 1.5 microns. Middle infrared is 1.5 to 5.6 microns. Far infrared is 5.6 to 1,000 microns. At this range, the invisible band of light warms objects, but not the air. The sun is an example. You can feel its warmth, even on a cold day. Approximately 80-percent of the sun's rays fall into an infrared range that penetrates your body anywhere from 1.5 to 3.5 inches. This is different from the harmful U.V. (ultraviolet) rays.

Microwaves are a group which are a horrible threat to human health. The strong electromagnetic waves of microwave radiation, when sub-jected to water or liquids which we may ingest as a warmed-up bever-age, destroys the beneficial vibrational crystalline frequency of life-giving water, as confirmed by specific studies. If we ingest microwaved liquids to replenish water lost by sweat therapy or exer-cise, we begin to resonate at the same damaged frequencies. This is certainly not good for health.

It should be noted that our own bodies radiate between 3 and 50 microns of infrared energy through the skin (recall the definition of radiation offered earlier). People who practice and use the Chinese healing art of qigong can actually emit this energy from the palms of their hands in the 8-14 micron range. This is something you can learn to do easily, as well, and is called *therapeutic qigong healing*. When you use FIR sauna, these healthy frequencies are absorbed into the body, and water in the cells respond with "resonant absorption." The frequency of the FIR matches the frequency of the water in the cells. The result: Toxins leave cells and enter the blood stream, then enter the organs of elimination which rid them from the body. Provided you don't overdo it, far infrared sauna use can be seen as giving yourself a self-induced qigong treatment. A person usually needs a qigong master to project these beneficial waves into his or her energy field.

Thus, with FIR sauna use, inflammation is created, internal heat is generated, and all the benefits of sauna therapy are gained. This is especially good to heal muscle injuries. The benefits of infrared sauna therapy are that less heat is necessary to produce the desired physiological effects. Benefits are gained by heating to 110°-120°F versus 150°-180°F in a normal sauna or steam sauna. While any type of sweat is better than "no sweat," another obvious advantage of FIR over steam is that if the water used in steam is not

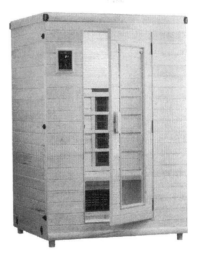

THERMAL LIFE® FAR INFRARED
2-PERSON POPLAR SAUNA
UNIT FROM HIGH TECH HEALTH, INC.
(800.794.5355)

pure (purified, filtered, reverse-osmosized, etc.), you will be taking in much of what you are trying to eliminate. Remember, you're breathing in the steam and it is coming back into your body through the opened pores. The impurities (fluoride, chloride, metals, chemicals) found in municipal water will find their way back, albeit in smaller amounts, into your system.

One aspect of FIR therapy, however, is that you have to be prepared for what might be a powerful detoxification. Based on dark field live blood cell, urine, and hair analysis, it appears that the infrared sauna produces a much more profound and rapid detoxification than other sauna sweat therapies. While it's a good thing, it is important to realize that the more toxic a body is, the more intense the detox will be. It's like the rush-hour crowd converging onto the subway for their ride home—it can be temporarily uncomfortable. It is important to supplement this detox with large amounts of liquids (filtered or alkalinized water is always a first choice); vitamins; minerals; enzymes; and toxin-neutralizing green drinks containing wheat grass juice, chlorella, spirulina, or barley grass — to help facilitate elimination, especially of heavy metals, during this stage. Our tests confirm this.

Another type of hyperthermia therapy is ultrasound. How this works is that high-energy sound waves are applied to the body. Friction is caused at the molecular level which generates heat. One application is sufficient for localized therapy, while, logically, multiple ultrasound heads are needed for whole-body therapy.

You may be inclined to ask at this point, Since heat therapy is so beneficial in prevention and treatment of disease, isn't there a way to have your cake and eat it, too, so-to-speak? Overheating the body makes you convulse and cooks your brain like pasta. If not enough heat is used, although even a little has great benefits, you may not eliminate or reduce the disease process sufficiently to be truly therapeutic. How can we have it both ways? In other words, is it possible to eliminate dis-ease with heat therapy without cooking ourselves to death in the process?

The answer to this may lie in what is called extra corporeal hyperthermia. It holds great potential in the future of disease treatment. An amount of blood is removed from the body, usually heated to 108°F, then re-introduced to the body. Recall what we said about the upper limits of the survival threshold of disease-causing entities? This is done in small increments of, perhaps, 100cc at a time. The heating process shows strong promise in the treatment of hepatitis—especially Hepatitis C which afflicts over 200 million people worldwide, HIV, other infectious diseases, and may even become additional therapy for cancer treatment.

The super-heating in this therapy, kills off invading organisms and what remains is clean, super-immune-charged blood going back into the body. After many treatments, a major part of the circulating blood volume has been treated and returned to the body in a much cleaner form. The blood and the patient are basically renewed and purified. And the best part is that the patient didn't have to experience the heat externally. Remember, 105°-106°F is a human body's upper-most limit.

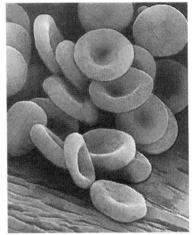

HEALTHY RED BLOOD CELLS

You would go into convulsions if your core temperature became this hot. This would be a classic case of "The surgery was a success, but the patient died!" This ultrasound therapy is similar to U.V.B therapy (ultra-violet B light) where blood is drawn, irradiated with the light in a device that looks like a small tanning chamber, then reintroduced to the body.

Now we reach the good old "do-it-yourself" therapy of exercise. While it may take some time to get to the hyperthermic sweat-inducing stage, exercise has numerous benefits to the body. Exercise has the potential to raise body temperature to between 102°-104°F. There is a surge of interest in heated yoga. This induces a massive sweat for about an hour to an hour-and-a-half, and provides a great muscle and cardiovascular workout. You may have to build up your tolerance gradually for the 100°F+ heat in the room; but once you do, you'll reap enormous benefits. Since yoga originated in India and most areas of India are hot, virtually all yoga done in India could be considered heated!

Qigong is another time-tested classic—and my favorite, as you can tell. This is yoga's close cousin and Chinese counterpart. There are numerous anecdotal accounts of people who live in extremely poor rural regions of China and India who were afflicted with life-threatening diseases and literally burned them out of their bodies by engaging in these arts, even without the benefits of adjunctive herbs or supplements, since many were too poor to even purchase these. Working up a good sweat caused them to generate internal fever, which killed off what ailed them. These types of exercises have been around for thousands of years, so are definitely not trends or fads.

I routinely practice qigong to bring my mind, body, and spirit into harmony. It is an indispensable part of my mental, spiritual, and physical training. Old qigong masters have given me long lectures on the quality of sweat attained through this practice. Sweat changes in character from the initial muscle activation phase of the exercise practice to a different taste, smell, and consistency as the qigong (or yoga) breathing assists inner organ massage which then pushes sweat out from the inner visceral organs to the skin. Toxins are sent out through all other detoxification channels, as well. A word of advice: Do some basic yoga or qigong to activate your inner organs prior to doing sweat therapy. This way, the activation of the nervous, cardiovascular, and endocrine systems make the detoxification even more effective. I realize I've mentioned this several times—because I know and experience the rewards of daily qigong practice—but these benefits are covered in my book, "Shaolin Yoga: Qigong" and my up-coming book, "Qigong Prescription."

While it can take a lifetime to master these exercises, one can easily learn them. Once you learn them, teach others. This can begin your journey to mastery. It is said in medicine, regarding procedures, "See one, do one, teach one!" And, if people think you are eccentric or going off on an eccentric (non-health-improving) tangent with these practices, remind them of The Roman Rule (also frequently cited in Chinese literature): "The one who says it cannot be done should never interrupt the one who is doing." I've had doctor friends ask me why I waste so much time training in these crazy things when I should just stay in my office and make money. Perhaps they are unfamiliar with the adage: "Health is wealth." By the way, one of these friends is now practicing "sound time-management techniques" by going to work whenever he can muster the energy between bouts of nausea and fatigue he experiences from chemotherapy treatments for his cancer.

Something else noteworthy: Based on personal observation, these practices expand and protect the protective layer of wei chi. If you recall, I explained that this is the protective interfacing bioenergy field around a person, sometimes called the aura. One particular morning when I felt rushed and did not take adequate time to bring my healing energy field into harmony, I worked on a patient who had advanced pancreatic cancer. This man was clinging to life, so naturally (but not visibly) clung onto my more powerful energy field. Just by mere chance, before he came into my office, I decided to look at my blood by doing a finger stick for a live blood cell analysis. My blood looked good and healthy. I treated my patient, checked his blood, and thought, "Why not check mine again?" This was about an hour after my original self-analysis. That's a relatively short period of time. I could not believe the change in my blood. My cells had developed a strange resemblance to that of someone with this type of cancer. I'd always believed this was a possibility, but this was my first time to observe it scientifically and verify it. It was a horrifying feeling, indeed. You may understand why I felt concern, and why I immediately did about 15 minutes of qigong ("Physician heal thyself" was taken seriously). After doing these exercises, I rechecked my blood and found it restored to its earlier healthy state.

This is why most doctors seem to have poor health and less vitality than most other people. If not the actual physical pathogens, they are certainly absorbing the bioelectrical negative energies of ill people they come in contact with. We know that most people visit doctors only when they are unwell. Since this is the level at which disease first develops, the implications are astounding. I'm now developing a course to teach doctors how to protect themselves bioenergetically from the sick energy of patients they are exposed to. As a doctor, this may, indeed, be my noteworthy contribution to the world of allopathic medicine! When people ask me where I get my seemingly boundless energy from, I tell them my physical, mental, and spiritual strength comes from my positive Zen attitude and purpose in life. I also add, "It's no sweat. Just know sweat!"

In short, please allow me, Dr. Bill, to say, "Don't sweat the problems, sweat the solutions!" Choose your own path or combination of detox therapies. Ask for advice if you're not sure what to do; but, ask it from a competent, knowledgeable person. Don't just think about it—do it. Emotion can be changed by motion, so start now. As Albert Einstein said, "Nothing happens until something moves."

"*Everybody's got the fever.*
That is something you all know.
Fever isn't such a new thing,
Fever started long ago.
Lyrics from "You Give Me Fever"
sung by Peggy Lee

SOME SWEATY COMPLICATIONS:
Complications of Fever

Anything can have complications, even sweat therapies; but, don't sweat it. Fever is a double-edged sword: It can heal and it can destroy—if abused. Fever induced recklessly and without proper knowledge and supervision can cause problems, even serious ones. It's important to know something about problems that can happen with uncontrolled, very high fever—and is why I recommend you consult with a health care provider or doctor who is experienced in these therapies. As in everything else, people with health issues should not shun sweat therapy, but approach it more gradually, with medical supervision, using more caution unless it is absolutely contraindicated by their condition. Several specific conditions are listed below.

Congestive Heart Failure (CHF)
CHF is the progressive failure of the heart as a pump. The most common indications are shortness of breath and swelling of the ankles. Prognosis is as bad as cancer. Many of these patients will die within five years unless profound measures are taken to control it (see the case histories in Chapter 12 for a different result when alternative methods were used). The intensely overloaded heart is so backed up with fluid, even ankle vessels swell. Regardless of the precipitating cause—heart disease; infection; poor quality of water, air, food; toxic

emotions; other toxins in the body—it usually does not have a favorable prognosis. Furthermore, the often-prescribed drugs to treat it—diuretics, digitalis-containing agents, anti-hypertensives, to name a few—build up as an unmetabolized soup to further toxify the already ailing organ. Subjecting a CHF patient to a rapid high-temperature sweat can kill him or her. Infrared sauna, with its low heat, used carefully and slowly, can help reverse this condition and restore health.

Convulsions
High, uncontrolled non-therapeutic fevers have been known to cause convulsions, no matter the age of the individual. Though more common in children, convulsions can happen in adults. The best treatment is prevention. In the domain of sweat therapy, a slow, methodic induction can prevent this. Knowing when to say When is the key. There is no room for heroics or macho attitude when it comes to sweat therapy. I have seen men in gyms try to outlast one another in steam rooms and saunas. This only leads to trouble. Your body knows when you've had enough. It is imperative that you listen to it. As you continue your sweat therapy routine, your endurance will improve and increase.

Delirium
The state of altered sensorium, once again, can occur by trying to take on too much temperature too fast.

Failure to Sweat
Congenitally missing sweat glands, a condition known as *anhydria*, prevents sweating. While this is a rare condition, **people born without sweat glands should definitely not use sweat therapy**. Anhidrosis, another term for decreased or non-existent sweating, can be life-threatening for some people. This may be a result of autonomic neuropathy (damage to nerves regulating the temperature), result from infections, burns, or dehydration. Often, it is a result of an inher-

ited condition. People with hypohidrotic ectodermal dysplasia (HED), a rare disorder, are born without sweat glands. This places them at a high risk of death from over-heating. A sure risk is allowing this type of child to participate in physically active, strenuous sports which would always cause a sweat in a normal child. These children will over-heat; and when the heat cannot dissipate, the results can be disastrous. Do not even let them look at a sauna door. Other detox protocols can be used by them such as colonic irrigation, juice fasting, and dietary modifications.

Certain conditions also inhibit a sweat response. For example, patients with advanced cancer, as indicated before, will usually not sweat at the start of these therapies no matter what we do. Cancer, in astrology, is symbolized by the crab. Cancer is, indeed, like a crab since it grabs on with its pincers and roots itself to the body. Once there, it exerts an autonomic effect on the body which represses the sweat function. With true patience and time, the patient can be made to sweat. I can tell you from experience, this is a very slow process.

Febrile Albuminuria
The export protein of the liver, called albumin, can be adversely affected by extremely high temperatures. Faulty production and breakdown occurs. This is seen in diseases of extreme fever. It is not a common finding in sweat therapy.

Headaches
A rapid dilation of cerebral arteries (increased intracranial pressure) may result in a headache. Again, slow acclimatization to heat will either reduce or eliminate headaches.

Hemophilia
Anyone with this condition must discuss sweat therapy thoroughly with their doctor. Sauna and other sweat therapies have the potential

to cause complications that should be avoided. This is a condition where other detox protocols should be explored.

Herpes Simplex Outbreaks

In certain circumstances, fever causes outbreaks when the virus is present and enacted in latent or active form, or can accentuate an outbreak. Outbreaks of a dormant herpes simplex virus have been reported on just about any area of the body. Although the exact mechanism is not defined, a very rapid detoxification may cause this.

Hyponatremia

This is discussed in Chapter 11 which focuses on athletes and performers—individuals whose jobs or activities cause them to sweat profusely. Unless totally abused, this condition is not a problem in therapeutic sweats.

Malignant Hyperthermia

This is an anesthesiologist's worst nightmare. While in the first year of my anesthesiology residency, one of our patients developed this while under anesthesia. The temperature shot up so fast, we had to pack ice in the patient's groin, armpits, and neck. The patient nearly died. A nursing student just lost it then-and-there. If I remember correctly, she changed specialties.

A rapid, uncontrolled rise in temperature will literally cook the brain unless the patient is immediately removed from anesthesia, given sodium dantrolene, and immersed in ice. While some cases have reportedly been induced by major stress, trauma, emotional upheaval, or strenuous exercise (with extreme heat production), the vast majority is limited to reactions from anesthetic agents. It is a disorder of muscle which effects body membranes, in general, and causes an immediate, intense rise in body temperature, muscle contractions, and convulsions. Unless you plan to go into anesthesiology as a career, don't worry too much about this one.

As a patient, unless there is a genetic predisposition in your family, don't get crazy about this. A simple muscle biopsy can be done to test for any such potential response to anesthesia.

Again, these explanations are not intended to scare you, just inform you. Many people read or hear the warning that they should consult with a physician or health care provider before starting an exercise or detox program—but they don't follow this advice. In general, a person who is considered healthy and just a bit toxic, should be able to exercise and do sweat therapy without any complications. People who know they have certain conditions or suspect they do, should get more information before the engage in any new protocol.

"Success is dependent upon the glands—sweat glands."
  Zig Ziglar

SOME SWEATY PRECAUTIONS AND GUIDELINES

Here are some precautions and guidelines to follow if you are going to engage in sweat therapy. Most of these are common-sense items, but I want to be sure to mention them in case any reader isn't certain about these specifics.

• Allow time before and after to enjoy the benefits. This should be your mental, physical, and spiritual detox time. Don't rush the experience. You're trying to reduce or release stress. Rushing through it because you have not planned enough time to do it properly is not the way to experience this. If you include any kind of stressor—poor scheduling, dwelling on problems or upsets, your body will do what it is designed to do: Release chemicals to answer your call for help. Then, you're defeating the purpose of this detox process because you're adding more chemicals that need to be eliminated and.... Well, if you've read every chapter up to this point, you know what I'm talking about. Since the body continues to sweat for at least 15-20 minutes after the sweat session is completed, sit in a relaxed environment, preferably wrapped in a towel or absorbent robe—or nude in a space where you won't get chilled, and appreciate the benefits of what you just did for yourself. As a rule, when the sweat coming out of your body smells totally neutral (no odor), the job is complete (the meat is well done, so no need to overcook!). Remember to include soothing music as part of this process, if that's possible. You might also research recordings of healing sounds that are available.

• Do not take alcohol for at least several hours before sweating (despite the Russian story told earlier). This will accelerate the assimilation, get you drunk, and defeat the purpose.

• Don't eat for a few hours before the sauna or sweat therapy. The energy expenditure that goes into digestion should go into detoxification and elimination. You don't want major organs and systems competing for your energy.

• Pre-prime your elimination system with some physical activity—yoga, qigong, tai chi, stretching, etc.

• Drink ample quantities of water before, during, and after—especially if you do two or three sweat sessions in a sequence. Since loss of salt, minerals, and electrolytes occur, supplementation with water is necessary. Ample does not mean to overdo water intake. You can literally drown if you drink too much. Chapter 11 goes into this in some detail.

• Use a scrub or do the dry-brush technique described earlier to remove dead skin. This will also activate the lymphatic channels, another major route described previously, to stimulate detoxification of toxins trapped in them. When you're done with your session, you want to remove any toxins on the skin, so either use a foaming body scrub that contains coarse particles or a different body brush, or the dry brush (but wash it off afterwards), and scrub down as you rinse off. Also, if you use your tub or home sauna, clean it after your session to remove toxins that adhere to the surface.

• Therapeutic oils and aroma therapy are excellent for improving your mood and physiology. You can typically find these at health food stores. And it's easy to learn which essences promote relaxation, such as lavender—a favorite. If your head is stuffy, use eucalyptus. There are almost always "experts" hanging around places that sell these essences, who will gladly and willingly give you guidance. But we are individual in our preferences, so find one or several that meet your needs.

• Chinese herbal essences such as kidney- and liver-enhancing teas will restore harmony to these organs. No reason you can't sip on a beneficial tea during the 15-20 minute interval. Doing so helps you sweat more readily. You might also want to explore the benefits of Bach Flower Remedies and Pegasus Products' Elixirs and Vibrational Remedies. I am coming out with a unique combination for this, myself.

• Don't be greedy. Wanting to sweat too much, too fast, with too much heat or prolonged exposure can only spell trouble.

• Use caution when the body has a high fever. It is better to use the sauna after the fever spikes and breaks in order to avoid hyperthermia. Sweat therapy should not be implemented during the acute, or febrile, phase of any condition.

• Use caution if you are fatigued or have not slept well. This diminishes your tolerance and causes excess vagal stimulation—vaso-vagal episodes are known as fainting. If you are pregnant, or on medications, or have a medical problem you are hesitant about, consult with your physician first.

• Supplemental doses of Vitamin B2—actually, all of the B-complex vitamins—will help. Vitamin E helps keep skin pliant. Ingestion of one of several herbs such as cayenne pepper, peppermint, ginger, and garlic, will promote sweating and keep the skin healthy. You can sprinkle cayenne pepper into your special tea to boost circulation and rev up sweating.

These are some primary things you should be aware of. If at any time during a sweat session you feel weak, stop the session. Sit quietly, sip water, and let your body cool off. It may be a response to the initial release of toxins into your blood stream or an initial response to unused-to heat or sweating—especially if you have been sedentary and rarely break a sweat. It could also be an indication of an imbalance in your body that prompts you to get a physical. Always heed your body's signals. It really does communicate messages to you. You just need to learn how to listen.

This is a good time for me to give you a relatively simple "Dr. Bill" protocol.

1. Make time to do this. This is a gift you give to yourself.

2. Relax; meditate; do tai chi, qigong, yoga, or just simple stretching for at least 15-20 minutes prior to your heat therapy. You want to get your chi (life energy) moving, massage your inner organs, and rev up your circulatory system to facilitate the detox process. Bring harmony to your mind, body, and spirit by listening to music that soothes and makes you feel good.

3. Drink some warm or hot tea. I highly recommend using Chinese herbal teas to boost the immune system. Watch for my new formulas coming out soon.

4. Drink two to three eight-ounce glasses of purified water (alkalinized is best) before, during, and after to stay hydrated.

5. Get into the sauna or sweat bath for 10-15 minutes. If you can do 20 minutes, do it. But you must listen to your body—and know that each session will be different. Remember, no macho attitude about this. It's not a competition, it's a healing session.

6. Remove yourself from the heat therapy. Drink another two to three eight-ounce glasses of water. Some massage at this point would be great; but if you don't have a private massage therapist on call, don't sweat it. Create some movement in your body any way that is comfortable to you.

7. Get back into the heat therapy for another 15-20 minutes.

8. Get out, drink more fluids as needed, but don't overdo the fluids at this point. Let the remainder of sweat, now much cleaner and less smelly at this point, leave your body. Don't rush to dress or do anything. Relax for this additional 15-20 minutes.

9. Shower and enjoy your day—or take a nap. If you do this treatment prior to going to bed for the night, enjoy your far-more restful, restorative sleep.

To use this for detox purposes, follow this protocol five to seven days a week. For simple maintenance, two to four times a week should be sufficient. You'll develop a healthy, hearty appetite sometime later. Don't forget to add minerals (I recommend Krystal Salt) to your food to replenish minerals you lost during the sweat.

Within one to two weeks, your friends will begin to notice a difference in the way you look. You'll notice not only an improvement in your appearance, but in how you feel.

Depending on your schedule, plan to do several sweat sessions as described above, back-to-back, whether once a week, once every two weeks, or once a month. You want to include what's been recommended so far (exercise prior to the sweat session, water and tea intake, etc.), but do two to three sessions in a row where you use the actual sauna or bath, rest for 10 to 20 minutes, then repeat. During the rest stage, it would be beneficial to give yourself a massage as best you can. Books on reflexology can teach you how to use this healthful technique on your feet and hands. Massage your legs, arms, torso, scalp, ears. Just as you should do during any sweat therapy session, focus on your intention. From the moment you begin the exercise part, release all thoughts that have nothing to do with where you are and what you are doing. Feel your body. Intend that your inner organs are receiving beneficial massaging. Intend that toxins are leaving your body. Intend that your internal and external body is in balance and radiantly healthy. If any conflicting thoughts about being healthy arise as you state your intentions to yourself, note them and give them genuine consideration later. One of the best things people can do for themselves is to look at the stories they tell themselves.

Ready to walk through the (sauna) door?

"I live every day to its fullest extent and I don't sweat the small stuff."
Olivia Newton-John

SOME SWEATY PROTOCOLS

By now, you may have worked up a sweat thinking about what happens if you don't sweat! Obviously, there is more to detoxifying the body than just getting rid of sweat, even though it's a huge cornerstone. By the end of this book, you'll be able to say **I Am Pure.** Let's use this as a mnemonic:

I - *Stands for intention.*
A - *Activation of your higher self and partnership with your body.*
M - *Mindfulness of new decisions that replace old ones that no longer serve you.*
P - *Purging of physical, mental, and emotional toxins-slowly, if necessary.*
U - *Undo damage with new lifestyle changes.*
R - *Repair and rebuild your body and reassure yourself that things can be reversed and that it's never too late!*
E - *Enjoy great health!*

When you make the decision to become truly healthy, a comprehensive mind-body-spirit program is the way to do it. People forget, or don't know, that they are holistic—or *Wholeistic*—beings. You can participate in the prevention and treatment of any imbalance or disease that affects your body. Begin with intention. Consciously intend to purify your body. A pure body will help maintain a pure mind.

I remind you of the quote I included earlier, "Treating a disease after it arises is like beginning to dig a well after you have become thirsty..." Dig your well now. I've said it before and will say it again (and again and again)—*disease is caused by toxin accumulations in the body.* These can be physical (internal or external), mental, or spiritual in nature. All can be dealt with, and best if dealt with simultaneously.

My book, *"Shaolin Yoga: Qigong,"* is a good introduction for how to follow this process. The content of this book facilitates the detoxification protocol by teaching proper breathing, activation of the higher self, and how to enter the *no mind* state—and why it is important to do so. The book also instructs on how to move correctly. Remember, "Motion can change emotion." This is a great first step.

You might believe that integrating protocols into your daily life is difficult in this high-stress technological lifestyle we have created; but, let me ask you—Was it any easier with plagues, minimal nutrition, famine, and wars going on over the last millennia or longer? Not really. See it all as easy, and so it must become. The quality of our environment has changed because of the Industrial Revolution, but we can contend with even this. In fact, it is imperative we do so if we wish to stay healthy. Our mental state and perceptions—how we react to problems—determine everything in our lives as positive or negative. Choose the positive. It is your right, as well as your responsibility to yourself, foremost. Why live sick and leave our planet early? Stick around for a while longer. Did you say you still have things you want to enjoy? Bungee jumping, race car driving, an enlivened sex life, and so forth? What about things you want to contribute to humanity?

We have to be realistic about the fact that it takes years to build up to a state of disease. Some of this is our doing. The remainder is just from living on our polluted planet. Therefore, you cannot expect to detox overnight. As Dr. Sherry Rogers puts it, "High-tech problems require high-tech solutions." Or, to use Einstein's quote, "No problem can be solved from the same level of consciousness that created it." If you try to speedily detoxify (society, especially in the work environment, places a high and misplaced value on speed), you risk creating additional problems you don't really want. If you engage in a detox program unwisely or unintelligently, you risk injury or even death. This is unnecessary.

You are now mindful, or mind full, of habits and toxins that are good ones to purge and eliminate. You know that a good place to start is with a knowledgeable physician or health care provider. Dr. Rogers' book, *"Detoxify or Die,"* strongly recommends some basic medical toxicity tests to give you a baseline of where you stand (Metametrix: 1.800.221.4640). This helps you scientifically understand how toxic your body is before you begin any protocol. (Also see www.lef.org.)

Now, I want to give you some tips and guidelines to consider for lifestyle recommendations and practices.

Water. Since we are what we eat and drink, make what you ingest as natural as possible. Drink eight to ten glasses of water per day. Water is responsible for every bodily function, including detoxification, and makes up about 70-percent of the body (more of lean body mass). You have to replenish thoroughly, every day. Undo, but don't overdo it, either. As I indicated before, **you can literally drown if you overdo water intake**. The recommended amount is sufficient. See Chapter 11 for examples of when you need more and how much more.

Avoid tap water as much as possible. Worried about simple survival, my parents never had water-filtering devices at home, just as I am sure many of you, as well, can't go back and change what happened previously. Just try to do your best going forward. As I indicated before, the body will take a lot of abuse before it unceremoniously tells or directs you where to go next. A study conducted by the National Resources Defense Council found that 18,500 of U.S. water systems (serving 45 million Americans) were in violation of safe-drinking laws at some point between 1994 and 1995. Despite the establishment of allowable limits, the Council's report blamed con-taminated water for 900,000 illnesses a year, including 100 deaths. Even if in small amounts, tap water contains harmful chemicals and inorganic minerals which are useless to the body. Water has been found to contain radon, fluoride, arsenic, iron, lead, copper, and other heavy metals. It may also have biological contaminants, pesticides, and other poisons. Don't think these haven't lodged into the deep lay-ers of your body. It's never too late to detox.

Referencing, again, the wisdom of Dr. Emoto, it's possible to influence and change the physical properties of water, for a time anyway, by pro-jecting positive thoughts and emotions at it. Emoto calls the life-giv-ing energy *Hado* (Tao). This is manifested in the change in the molec-ular bonding of the water by affecting the electrons' and protons' orbits. This, ultimately, affects the bond angle between the hydrogen molecules, which are normally 104.45 degrees. This affectation can be influenced by external or internal negatives or positives. When we project positive energy into water prior to drinking it, we get super-charged water, even if it wasn't the best water to begin with.

One or more people can do this to food or water, akin to the blessing offered by many before a meal, which holds implications of increased health and serenity going into the body via what it ingests. Since microscopic confirmations validate this result, this moves it out of "new age" rhetoric into scientific experiments that can be duplicated. Dr. Emoto also found that poisonous or toxic polluted water never forms the natural, beautiful crystals unless radical bioenergetic measures were taken to restore it. Tragically, the most important healthful fluid needed by the human body (and all organic organisms) is becoming polluted in ways never seen by humanity to date.

After this, the next step is to purge. If you are going to detoxify and purge toxins from your body, it makes sense to limit the toxic substances you put into your body and bring in the main vehicles which will help carry them out. Water is a good place to start. Aim for purified, reverse-osmosis treated or alkalinized water (alkaline water machine). A pH reading of seven is neutral. Reverse osmosis water has a pH of 6.6, a far cry better than tap water and far cleaner. Alkalinized water has a 9.6pH reading. Recall that a low pH (acidic) and low-oxygen environment is conducive to disease. Bacteria, viruses, other germ-causing agents, and cancers love a low pH, low-oxygen environment. It's where they thrive, so don't give them the chance. You can get an alkalinizer from High Tech Health International.

Rebuild with **Good Food**. It is often difficult to grow one's own food in this day and age. It is best to eat organic or kosher foods whenever possible. It is also important to learn what the different levels of "organic" mean. Don't assume that because a food is labeled organic that it is 100-percent so, not even if purchased at a health food store. Become informed.

Unfortunately, most foods are irradiated by the time they get to you. This alters their natural healing frequencies and can cause these foods to be harmful. While you would not want a poisonous tropical spider hanging out in the bunch of bananas on your kitchen counter, and even though irradiation kills bacteria and pathogens, it is harmful to food.

If you eat meat, fish, poultry, eggs, or cheese, aim for animals raised in a free-range environment, as well as raised on proper feed that did not include growth hormones, antibiotics, or other unnatural chemicals or substances. Know that the darker the color of fruits and vegetables, the higher the antioxidant properties (ORAC). If you're sensitive to mold, avoid melons and nuts. Many people misunderstand the whole topic of carbohydrates. There are simple and complex carbohydrates. Fruits and vegetables are complex carbohydrates, and are the ones you want. Learn which fruits produce sugar-level spikes and avoid them, as well.

You can choose to be monastic about what you ingest, but you really don't have to go that far unless you want to. If you are healing an imbalance or disease, you probably should adhere to only the proper foods until you've regained your health. Otherwise, pick a day when you will indulge in some of the other foods like certain desserts. Health is about balance. If you do more of the right stuff—proper food choices, adequate water intake, detox protocols such as sweat therapies, enough restful sleep and periods of relaxation, and exercise— you'll experience the well-being you seek. The body is designed to repair and rebuild itself. You just need to be willing to give it what it needs to do so. Remember the mnemonic: I Am Pure!

Dr. Gabriel Cousens has written a wonderful book on spiritual nutrition called, *"Spiritual Nutrition and the Rainbow Diet."* He states, as many healers have in the past, that to practice spiritual nutrition, one must take in just the right amount of food and drink according to our individual needs. Our bodies, which are really "mature crystals," function within the physical laws of crystals at the very intricate level, can be harmonized; and the core energy, referred to as kundalini, can be spiritualized. There is a constant "transmutation" of energy. Since the plant, animal, and human kingdom are so closely linked, the laws of "biologic transmutation," plant blood—magnesium-containing chlorophyll—can become transmuted to iron-containing hemoglobin, the oxygen and life-carrying component of blood (theory of biologic transmutation). Just as you try to avoid acid-producing (negative) emotions, limit at the least, acid-producing foods. You want your body to be more alkaline than acidic. This should be practiced along with right thought, speech, and action which, of course, leads to right livelihood.

The downside of truly purifying yourself with all the techniques I've given you, is that you may, on many levels, become sensitive to environments which are polluted—conditions that don't seem to bother persons who are as polluted, or nearly so, as the environment. This is why finding balance and avoiding either extreme is vital to your well-being.

If you decide to give more conscious attention to what you ingest, make it an inward journey. Every food group has a vibrational energy which has been designed to work in synergy with the vibrational energy in your chakras—the energy centers in your body. The color and frequency of these two should be matched to ensure maximum benefit.

If someone asks why you look better than ever and seem to have more energy, tell them something about what you're doing, perhaps recommend this book to them; but don't try to convert them or appear judgmental about their habits. This kind of behavior not only comes across as intrusive, but always backfires because no one wants to feel judged. Unless you've decided to be compulsive about it, go to restaurants with friends and choose foods wisely. It's really unnecessary to engage the waiter with questions about whether or not the water is filtered or if the food is organic. You can either choose to eat at organic restaurants or choose to enjoy a meal with a friend at a restaurant of his or her choice. To carry on about all of this when your friend believes you are going to share quality, relaxing time together spoils the moment and affects the digestive process. For everyone.

Also, take a moment to appreciate good food and those whose efforts went into its provision. Appreciate the wonder of your body's digestive and assimilation abilities. Appreciate the well-beingness that comes from good foods, good times, and good friends. Meals are times of appreciation, not times for arguments, break-ups of relationships, or negative conversations. Meals are like meditation or prayer. Good mental and spiritual chi will lead to good digestive chi. Think negative thoughts during meals, and everything from digestion to assimilation and elimination will be affected. Mealtimes should be honored for what they are.

Do not underestimate the importance of rest to rebuild your system. This cannot only spiritually enhance you through dreams, but will allow you to extract maximum nutrients from your foods. This was briefly mentioned in the section on stress. Taoist monks living in ancient China, systematically categorized the cycles of organ systems and their optimal time of function. They came to recognize, without the help of high-technology, that most of the assimilation cycles occur during the waking hours while the breakdown—degradation and cleansing—takes place in the wee hours of the morning. That is, the internal organs involved with these functions and their associated flow and distribution channels (meridians) are most active between 10P.M. and 6A.M. These are the liver, gall bladder, and large intestine. For this reason, sleep had between the hours listed here, appears to be most beneficial to the human body. It is a rebuilding rest for the body. More research needs to be done concerning persons who work jobs that involve reverse circadian rhythms, i.e., police officers, nurses, night-shift workers, etc., since the change from nighttime sleep (when it's dark) to day (when it's light) undoubtably takes a toll on health in the long-term.

Colonics. This is a good way to cleanse the body as it has multiple benefits. A condition called *leaky gut syndrome* is where minute particles of undigested or partially-digested food passes through the swollen or inflamed mucosal wall of the colon. This can cause allergic reactions and can be mitigated by cleaning out this organ of elimination. Sweat therapy, although it possesses numerous benefits, can drive toxins out through the skin, but also through other organs such as the colon. A clean, functional colon, cleared of years of accumulated toxic waste, helps you eliminate faster and better. You can do your own oral colonic therapy using bentonite or psyllium husk products—if you haven't gotten over the anal stage (most never get over the oral stage, as well!).

You can even do an oral salt-water colon cleanse. This is easy and inexpensive, but you truly need to allow for four uninterrupted hours near a bathroom. Add two level teaspoons of uniodized sea salt, or Krystal salt to a quart of lukewarm water. Mix well and drink. It may take up to one hour to get going (or less), but it cleans your colon top-to-bottom. It flushes out plaque, gunk, and parasites. [See *"Prostate Health in 90 Days (without drugs or surgery)"* by Larry Clapp, Ph.D., J.D. This excellent book also gives, in some detail, the link between dental health (microbes found in the oral cavity) and illness in the rest of the body.] If you have high blood pressure, consult with your physician first. Plan time to follow this cleanse with sweat therapy to remove excess salt from your body.

Colonic irrigation is a great way to clean out the system in conjunction with sweat therapy. It may seem strange to voluntarily allow someone to put a tube into the rectum and remove waste, but it's useful. For those who've never done this, let me give you some information before you run down to a colonics center or provider, unaware of what is involved. You *will* have a tube inserted into your rectum. The facilitator *will* be there with you, engaging in conversation as you both watch fecal matter being removed and moving through a strange-looking contraption that looks like a modified cappuccino machine. For those of us still "stuck" at the anal stage of development, you may have to, psychologically, work up to this. Believe me, the results are worth it. However, if this image is uncomfortable for you, do the oral colonics mentioned in the above paragraphs. I recommend a colon cleanse at the change of each season to acclimatize the body to the new season, the seasonal foods, and any new emotions you experience.

A parasite cleanse is a must if you want a clean body. Colonics will achieve a good part of it, but not all. If you have traveled to any tropical area; eaten any form of meat, vegetables, fruit; or drink tap water, You Have Parasites! Parasites not only deplete your essential vitamins, minerals, and other vital trace elements, they poop out a toxic waste product, as noted before, that disrupts metabolic pathways (Dr. Hulda Clark). These toxic residues deplete the body of oxygen and create an acidic (low pH) environment. This sets up the foundation for cancers and other killer diseases. Colon cleansing, colonics, irrigation cleansing, and diet protocols—along with sweat therapy—help you rid your body of these nasty creatures. Prune seed extract, grapefruit seed extract, and therapeutic teas should help you undo the rest. These creatures also seem to dislike pumpkin seeds.

My constant travels to remote areas of the world to provide medical and dental goodwill work, often has me returning home having picked up many uninvited guests in my body until I detox them out with cleanses, Chinese herbs, and oxygenation and sweat therapies. In these travels, I also run into some fascinating people—which invariably off-sets the nuisance re-acclimation to an environment that's perhaps, at least, a bit more parasite-free. While in Tibet, the head doctor showed me manuscripts, with text I later verified through different books, that outline and categorize the presence of over 2,000 different types of bacteria and parasites in great detail. These were provided by the old great master—Buddha, himself—over 2,500 years ago, without the benefit of microscopes. Once again, as I always say, science just confirms what was intuitively known. Where science ends, faith begins. The domain of the (still) unknown.

If you truly wish to cleanse and get well, do a gall bladder/liver cleanse. A lymphatic cleanse also helps rid waste out of the body's lymphatic, or natural filter system. A knowledgeable body-work or massage therapist can help with this. Qigong and yoga also assist this process in a natural way. Dr. Paavo Airola gives some wonderful protocols in his excellent book, *"How to Get Well."*

Breath. Fresh air that is well-assimilated is integral for healing disease. Air chi, along with food chi, genetic chi, and environmental chi is considered a cornerstone of general heath by Indian and Chinese healing sages. Without proper breathing and oxygenation, the body cannot burn and assimilate food properly. To do so in a contaminated environment is counter-productive, to say the least. Generally speaking, mountains and ocean regions have good chi. The combination of both is ideal. It is helpful, and advised, that you learn to breathe like a Taoist monk. Proper breathing happens at the abdominal level—the diaphragm—rather than in the chest. If you aren't familiar with this, lie down, relax into a state of calmness and notice that it is your abdomen (diaphragm) that rises and falls, not your chest and shoulders. You can use this breathing style as part of your sweat therapy. Just do so carefully. Breathe the heat into the inner organs to help the detox process be more effective. These are slow, deep breaths; not rapid, shallow ones.

Fasting. This is one of the least expensive, easiest, and effective ways to detoxify and a great addition to sweat therapy. In a fast, you eliminate the intake of new toxins while you break down old ones, lower the body's workload, improve the immune system, lower the energy needed for food digestion—which involves the use of blood, oxygen, and nutrients and, thereby, help every system in the body. You literally shift the body's energy from daily routines so it diverts energy to cleaning itself up. Fasting also has a strong spiritual component. It improves a person's awareness and sensitivity and is used to supplement spiritual practice in many cultures. There are different types of fasts: Water, juice, and different combinations, thereof. It is a good idea to do an initial one-day-a-week fast, 24-hours in duration, for beginners. Once the body is strengthened sufficiently, a 48- to 72-hour fast can be tolerated. A 4- to 5-day fast once a year is an incredible cleansing mechanism when used with sweat therapy. An excellent book on this subject is by Paul C. Bragg, *"The Miracle of Fasting."* Choose a day or days when you don't have to work and can relax or go outside. Don't try to fast and focus at the office if you're not used to fasting. Also, if you have a serious health issue, please check with a knowledgeable health care provider before deciding to fast.

A word of caution about fasting: The body, when starved, first starts to break down carbohydrates for energy. The liver is mobilized. The next source is fats, then proteins. At the protein breakdown stage, we see major irreversible, life-threatening conditions associated with breakdown of organs and fluid build-up (ascites) with swollen bellies and, ultimately, a catastrophic outcome called *kwashiorkor*. We have seen photos and films of this in developing countries such as Africa, where children look like stick figures with bellies swollen with fluid. I want to briefly climb onto my soap-box and say the natural and controlled food resources of this planet are so abundant, there can only be one reason anyone starves or lacks any basic needs—someone's agenda. End of lecture.

In a non-starvation fast, we encounter some very interesting physiological changes, especially in the fat-breakdown segment. When fats are degraded to become energy for the body in the second stage, what gets released into the body? You know the answer as well as I do. Biological toxins, pesticides, chemical food additives, heavy metals, and everything the body has managed to store in the fat tissues to protect itself. The body can detoxify only so much out of its toxic "garbage dump" at a given time. While it is dangerous to carry these toxins around in fatty and other tissues, a rapid release of toxins into the blood via fasting without some detoxification and elimination protocol, may be dangerous to your health. A juice fast, at least in the initial stages of a fast, is preferable. Detoxifying herbs, minerals, and Chinese herbal teas are helpful to bind and eliminate these toxins. You need to push them out not only through the normal waste-product paths, but through the skin as sweat. Sweat therapy during a fast is not a luxury, it is a necessity if you truly wish to clean out your body. Just be sure to follow the guidelines and precautions I've provided, especially if you feel faint or exhausted from the release of toxins stored in your tissues.

Weight loss and crash diets. It is important to not carry around more weight than our skeletal structure was designed to optimally carry. You can find people who experience knee and foot problems, yet do nothing to reduce the extra 50, 100, or more pounds they demand their skeletal structure attempt to hold up. If you carried that much weight, like a large boulder, every moment except when sitting or lying down, you'd wear out in no time. This is why I propose a holistic approach to health. There really is no magic bullet. It takes conscious effort. Obviously, there is more involved than just over-eating when people carry far more weight than they should. Obesity is a seriously compromised, toxic environment. Quality of health and life are depleted. One reason people who are obese sweat so readily is their bodies are desperately attempting to detoxify.

People who jump from diet to diet or from over-eating to dieting or fasting, trigger the release of toxins from fat tissues which are constantly being broken down, and disrupt normal metabolism. Weight loss is nearly impossible when the body is toxic because the normal pathways of elimination are disrupted. Some medications cause weight or fluid gain, which indicates what they are doing to the rest of the body as they attempt to deal with an imbalance or disease. If you wish to lose weight, approach this methodically and gradually. Rapid weight loss is just unhealthy.

There is also something of an epidemic in the business world. Some have decided that the way to impress those at the top is to work non-stop at warp speed for three-quarters or more of each day; to keep a serious countenance on their face and in the way they hold their bodies; and to either eat while they work, delay meals by hours, or miss them entirely. If you've read every word in this book up to this point, you know this example says that there are people who agree to throw any sense of balance for work, rest, and play out of their lives; hold their bodies in stiff, rigid postures; increase their toxic levels, and throw their metabolisms off—so they look good at the office. Jobs don't kill us, as a rule; our agreement to compromise our health kills us. We agree to it. Amazing.

Supplements

There are many resources on the subject of supplements. This is not a complete nutrition book by any means, but I'll give you some guidelines here. I do encourage you to do research and become somewhat expert about these. There are several I feel are important to mention, along with nutrional tips, that help detox and strengthen the body:

Aloe Vera Juice. A great internal cleanser and purifier, as well as a proven external facilitator of healing.

Apples. Organic apples, whenever accessible, are a great source of nutrition, natural Vitamin C, quercetin—an antioxidant, and pectin—which binds heavy metals.

Avocado. This delicious fruit is a rich source of glutathione which is a major free radical fighter. Glutathione levels decrease as we age. It combines with fat-soluble toxins, especially alcohol, to make them water soluble and easily eliminated. Anyone who drinks has probably had an occasion to experience a hangover. Heavy drinking consumes glutathione; so, enjoy lots of guacamole with your margaritas.

Beet Root. A very potent blood purifier that absorbs heavy metals and is an excellent source of methionine which binds to waste products and removes them from the body.

Chlorophyll. Foods that contain chlorophyll are excellent for you. They are great immune system builders and detoxifiers for the human body. You can buy liquid chlorophyll at a health food store (even offered with natural mint flavoring). Chlorophyll is to a plant what blood is to mammals. The only difference is that the central atom is magnesium versus iron in human blood. Therefore, it is possible to build good, pure blood via the theory of biologic transmutation by taking in lots of chlorophyll. In fact, don't hesitate to add a capful to every glass of water you drink daily. Plant blood can actually be transformed into human blood through this complex reaction. If this were not so, vegetarians would die. Since red blood cells carry oxygen and white blood cells fight off disease, we want plenty of this in our system. If you've ever had a dog or cat, you've seen them eating blades of grass. They use their sense of smell to pick just the right blades, then nibble until they get enough. Intuitively, they know they need it.

Cruciferous Vegetables. This is the group that contains cabbage, brussels sprouts, spinach, kale, and cauliflower. These contain glucosinolates which induce the liver to produce vital enzymes. They are rich in indole (also spelled indol) carbonic acid, considered one of the most powerful disease-fighters of all time. The actual chemical component is Indole 3-Carbonol. This is a great discovery. Indoles are health-protecting, immune system-boosting plant-growth regulators that play an important role in clinical diagnostics and microbiology. They should be taken as part of every sound nutritional program, whether in vegetable- or capsule-form, which provides an equal level of protection against disease. Indoles that belong to this group have an unbelievable effect in preventing and reversing hormone-related tumors such as breast and cervical cancers, as well as many other types of cancers. Researcher Maria Bell refers to studies indicating elimination of even third-stage hormone-related cancers such as uterine cancers, with the use of Indole Carbonic Acid. It is a must. Note: People recovering from hypoadrenia are often advised to forego eating cruciferous vegetables for the duration of treatment. Check with your health care provider on this.

Garlic. Not just to keep away vampires (basically parasites of a different kind). Add this to your food and you can leach out toxins such as heavy metals, food contamination pollutants, and other hormonal break-down products. Garlic contains allicin, a sulfur-based compound. All bio-chemical reactions are based on these sulfur bonds. Sulfur keeps the body alkaline, and you recall what the benefits of this are. Garlic can help prevent disease and kill off most parasites. It creates a hostile environment for them as does grapefruit seed extract. Note: Some medications, even Chinese herbs, advise that you eliminate grapefruit from your diet while using the drug or following a protocol. Check the literature that comes with the drug or herbal protocol. Also, a good indication of parasitic load in the body is to look for dark circles under the eyes. They will sap your chi, or life energy. Parasites are not the only cause of this, but people with parasites usually do have dark circles there. So those of you who spend money on topical products to reduce this, consider getting rid of those dark circles by ridding your body of vital-energy-sapping parasites. Fresh garlic is best, but it still retains most of its benefit when cooked. For those who are averse to the taste or odor, its benefits can still be obtained in supplement form.

Green food products and supplements. Fresh wheat grass juice is a great detoxifier and blood cleanser. Any green food product will bind to toxins, including heavy metals. Green Magic™ manufactured by New Spirit Naturals, is an excellent one. Chinese parsley (cilantro) is an excellent heavy metal detoxifier, as is watercress. Nature's most concentrated forms of these one-cell food chain organisms are spirulina, chlorella, barley grass, and blue-green algae. All are indispensable dietary health supplements.

High Orac Foods. Orac is a measure of oxygen radical absorption capacity—the ability to break down free radicals. This is one of the most exciting concepts to be developed in the last decade. Orac foods are those dark-colored fruits like plums and their dried forms— prunes, blueberries, strawberries, blackberries, pomegranates, etc. The darker the fruit, the higher the orac value and the greater the potential to detoxify and rebuild.

Seaweed and Kelp. These contain high doses of iron, iodine, calcium, and magnesium. The alginates in seaweed help the body bind and eliminate toxins. Also, these are excellent to consider in the management of thyroid disease. Because of its high iodine content, this rejuvenates the thyroid gland which can be affected by radiation, toxins, and other substances. Note: Some people are sensitive to iodine. And, people with Hepatitis C are often advised to monitor their iron intake, including either limiting or eliminating iron pots and skillets for cooking. Again, check with your health care provider.

Toxin-Binding Foods. Kiwi, alfalfa, asparagus, carrots, bananas, eggs, and bran.

Vitamins, Minerals, and Other Goodies

Sweat therapy does create some stress for the body, but if done properly, this induced stress is a good stress. Nutritional support helps you maximize your detox process. It also allows you to rebuild your body afterwards. We are seeing an accelerated assault on the supplement industry. Conflicting reports exist that state vitamins are not effective and may even cause harm. This may (possibly) be valid, to some degree, for artificial (synthetic) ones. In case you aren't aware of this, pro-pharmaceutical industry lobbyists are desperately trying to pass legislation called CODEX. This legislation is designed to put supplements in the hands of licensed doctors. Become aware of this threat to the supplement market.

As a doctor with a wide range of experience in many healing modalities, from allopathic to Chinese medicine, it is my belief that proper choices and amounts of vitamins and minerals are essential to good health. Our food and water sources are simply too compromised to provide all that we need. When we detoxify our bodies, it is important to keep these levels in their optimal ranges. As far as **minerals** are concerned, I will go into these in a future book; but the major minerals to use to keep in balance are boron, calcium, chromium, copper, germanium, iodine, iron, magnesium, manganese, molybdenum, phosphorus, potassium, selenium, silicon, sulfur, vanadium, and zinc. Some are needed in trace amounts, so watch the dosages. In other words, don't over-do it. A great source of minerals is Krystal Salt.

There are many mineral complex preparations on the market to choose from. My advice about whether or not to take vitamins and minerals: Use your own judgment.

One good way to determine if something is good for you is to do a kinestetic test. You need one other person to help with this. One person holds something they know is unhealthy for them in one hand, and raises that arm to shoulder-level. The other person presses, not forcefully, down on the arm. Both observe how far the arm moves. The same person holds something they know is healthy for them in the same hand and the process is repeated. What this shows us is that when something is beneficial for you, your arm maintains strength. When it is not beneficial, your arm—often to the surprise of the holder—cannot maintain the same strength. An amazing testament to the energetic connection of people is when this test is performed with multiple individuals, say three or four, and the one at the far end of the link smokes a cigarette, the energy of the person on the opposite end is weakened merely by holding hands in the line. Each individual physiology is unique. Do not assume that because something is good for someone else it is good for you. Listen to your body.

Vitamin A is a powerful free radical-destroying detoxifier. It reduces the oxidation of DNA and disables reactive oxygen species, preventing damage to skin, lungs, and eyes. Do follow the recommended dosage since high doses may interfere with normal control of cell division. Note: Vitamin A applied topically to blemishes or acne, clears up the affected area(s).

B Vitamins are important cleansers. They help rid the intestinal tract of metals and improve nervous system function.

Vitamin C (Ester C) at 3,000-10,000mg daily, will help remove toxins and heavy metals from the body and, of course, free radicals. It is a potent antioxidant. This is at the very top of the list. Linus Pauling, the great scientist and Nobel Prize winner, reportedly took over 25,000mg per day! He lived well into his nineties. When he was diagnosed with prostate cancer, people said, "See! You took all those vitamins and still got cancer." His reply was, "Well, if I hadn't taken them, I probably would have gotten prostate cancer in my fifties or sixties or earlier." Another trailblazer. Poor soul was under the assault of the legal and medical system his whole life, like all pioneers. Just look at the legacy he left. I know he followed this protocol, but I don't know if he tried any other protocols over his lifetime or at the time of his illness.

Vitamin E at 400-800IUs per day is recommended as a powerful antioxidant that prevents the oxidation of lipids (fats). It protects cell membranes, improves circulation, and prolongs the life of red blood cells.

Alpha Lipoic Acid and **R-Lipoic Acid** are detoxifiers and heart protectors, and should be used regularly. Used along with a carnotine and carnosine extract, noted before, this makes a beneficial anti-aging combination. Add Coenzyme Q-10 to this mix, and you've got quite a combination, indeed. The Life Extension Foundation has a very good line of these and is also a great source of wisdom for general health and well-being. You can contact them and use the code "CFH" (as in Center for Healing) to get access to these health-enhancing formulations.

Coenzyme Q-10 and **Coenzyme A** are so powerful, you should make them not only a part of your detox program, but part of your life-extension program, as well. These are oxygen enhancers which boost immune system function. They protect cells and enhance heart function. They are also great for gingival (gum) health and protection. Taking 200-500mg a day is okay for a healthy person. The dose can be increased when disease is present.

Digestive Enzymes, when taken on an empty stomach, vacuum the body of its junk. These have been called the "sparks of life" by the late Dr. Edward Howell, a pioneer in enzyme research. They are essential for every life function from digestion, to assimilation, and repair. The three main categories of digestive enzymes are amylase, protease, and lipase. Also, don't forget to include the free radical-scavenging groups of metabolic enzymes known as superoxide dismutase (SOD) and counterpart, catalase. SOD is an antioxidant that attacks and neutralizes a common health-destroying free radical, superoxide. Catalase breaks down hydrogen peroxide, a metabolic waste product, and liberates oxygen. We discussed how beneficial a well-oxygenated environment is to the body. This is probably one of the most exciting frontiers in medicine. When these enzymes cannot find food to break down, it is believed they get to work on toxins and bad cells in the body, such as cancer. The protein and lipid coats of these bad cells are readily attacked and destroyed by these and other immune-fighting cells. You can literally help the body eat its way to health. This is far easier on the body than chemotherapy. Since the body rids itself of minerals and trace elements with sweat, as well as through everyday living, take adequate amounts of a mineral complex, as well.

Supplementation of the intestines with **good bacteria** (acidophilus and bifidus), especially after a colon cleanse, is a good way to restore colonic function, as well. I may be partial to Chinese medicine, but I've seen enormous benefits with the use of Chinese herbal teas. Teas that help clean out toxins from the system and rebuild liver and kidney chi are also very helpful.

Glutathioine (with L-Methionine and L-Cystine) is needed for its sulfur properties. It is a potent antioxidant that inhibits formation of free radicals and protects the body from their damage. Its major impact is on heavy metals and toxins.

Lecithin helps rebuild brain and other nervous system tissue and protects the nervous system from heavy-metal poisoning.

Omega-3 and **Omega-6** (essential fatty acids) cannot be manufactured by the body and are basic building blocks essential to most bodily functions, as well as immune system protection. Examples are fish oil, flaxseed oil, primrose oil, evening primrose oil, and grapeseed oil.

Vibrational Remedies

The infinite wisdom of nature can now be purchased, if you will, in a bottled and packaged form. Long before any commercial preparation and merchandising processes were invented, there were ancient healers who intuitively understood and knew the healing power of nature, which resulted in formulations to address specific organ systems. These were made available to the public on a wide scale thanks to the pioneering efforts of Dr. Edward Bach of England. This great physician and thinker started out as an orthodox (standard) physician, but realized that stress, emotions, and specific disease states have a powerful link. Attuned to the subtle energetic resonance of plants, Bach eventually left his practice and moved to the English countryside to dedicate his life in isolation so as to focus his attention on capturing the subtle energies of nature which led to his development of Bach Flower Remedies. He discovered that essences of certain flowers affected him, so why wouldn't they affect others similarly in these positive ways. He collected and painstakingly categorized flowers and steeped those identified to have certain bioenergetic frequencies that harmonized dysfunctional energetic patterns associated with illnesses and imbalances. He allowed the flowers to sit in pure water, left in sunlight, and discovered the energy of the plants transferred to and was retained in the physical properties of the water.

The specific bioenergy of particular flowers resonated with the physical body and countered negative emotions at the biofreqency level. When left untreated, the person ultimately developed an associated disease. As an example, he used impatiens flower extraction to treat people who felt irritable and impatient. An alcohol preservative was used to maintain the healing frequency passed onto the water. Eventually, he developed 38 essences. The 38th one is one of the most popular of the remedies—for good reason—and is known by the name "Rescue Remedy." Advocates keep this on hand for when extremely stressful conditions arise in life.

Another vibrational energy sage, Gurudas, followed suit by capturing the vibrational imprint not only of flowers, but of gems (gem elixirs), which he used to affect bodies physically and bioenergetically. He created 108 new flower essences that were categorized by those affecting the physical body in one group and the emotional body in another group. In both groups, changes at the specific meridian and chakra levels were believed to be induced.

Homeopathy, developed by Samuel Hahnemann as mentioned before, was the actual form of practiced medicine in the U.S. prior to 1900. The Flexner Act changed the way medicine was taught and utilized, and virtually eliminated homeopathy as a form of healing. In the early 1800s, this brilliant German physician became disenchanted with the "standard" of health care at the time and by coincidence, discovered through experimenting on himself (like many scientists, myself included) that symptoms of malaria (intermittent fevers) could be induced by taking, ironically, enough of a substance (chincona) traditionally used as a cure for the disease. He originated the "Law of Similars"—like cures like. Homeopathic remedies were developed based on their ability to reproduce the patient's "total complex of symptoms" in people who were otherwise healthy. Thus, strep throat could be treated by isolating the bioenergy obtained from the offending bacteria, streptococcus. The actual bacteria held the cure. (Sort of like taking a shot of the "hair of the dog that bit you.")

Homeopathic solutions are similar to flower remedies in that the actual solution contains not a single molecule of the original herb or flower. The process of progressively diluting the solutions maintains the bioenergetic imprint of the original substance captured by the energy-capturing medium—again, the highest energy-encompassing medium of earth and life—water. In the practice of homeopathy, less is more. The more diluted a substance, the more powerful its effects. The remedy matches the frequency of the emotion or illness, which refracts it and, thereby, causes the identical symptoms of the disease to manifest and, thus, eliminate it from the body by helping the immune system activate and build resistance to it. I have used vibrational frequency-enhanced ozone—another form of matter capable of capturing and retaining energy—to remove particular parasites from my body, probably picked up on my medical mission work in third world countries.

Because of my love of the Chinese culture and Chinese medicine, I am truly blessed to have met my spiritual brother, Dr. James Zhou, who was given sacred centuries-old formulas from his Taoist monk teachers. He has given me the education and the formulas to use so that others may benefit. Our combined "centuries" of experience in various healing modalities and Chinese medicine, resulted in the creation of vibrational-enhanced tinctures used as teas. These are a great addition to any detox protocol and general diet.

Life-Saving Protocols

No one likes the word diagnosis—especially when it's attached to a life-threatening disease. It is so definitive, so permanent. It attaches the disease to your body's spirit and soul. You become the disease. It is you and you are it. One of my medical school professors once seriously asked our class if anyone knew what the biggest cause of death was. We shouted out the usual names of diseases you might imagine. None of us got it right. He finally shocked the entire class by saying—"Being born!" Without wanting to get into a political debate about this, you can say that either from the moment of birth or the moment of conception, we begin the process of dying.

In eulogies, there is a dash between the birth date and the death date. There are many opinions on this that include that a life span is predetermined by the creator one believes in, decided before birth by the individual, or the luck of the draw. We have many beliefs about this, but no empirical evidence. What we do have is an opportunity to do all we can to participate in the quality and quantity of the time period represented by the dash. Jim Morrison, lead singer of The Doors, said, "Nobody gets out of here alive."

Just as there are many beliefs about the life span, there are also many beliefs about why we are born. Death is a natural cycle of life. Many stories are told on this subject. Religious books, undoubtedly, have tons of ideas and theories and supposed facts on this. One story I particularly love, and probably originated somewhere in the Middle East, is about a man walking in a bazaar who gets tapped on the arm by a person wearing a hooded cape. Not able to see the man's face, the visitor asks, "Do I know you?" The mysterious character replies, "No, but my name is Death and we have an appointment tomorrow morning at six o'clock." Panic-stricken and paralyzed by fear, the man uses all his savings to buy three horses, food and water, then sets out to outrun his destiny, wanting to put as much distance between himself and "Death" as possible. He rides hard through the desert that night, exhausting each horse one-by-one. Finally, believing he has beat his curse, he arrives at a watering hole, weary and thirsty, as is his horse. He sees a lone soul sitting there. This individual turns around and looks at the man and says, "Incredible," and looks at his watch. "I never thought you'd make it in time." Thus, despite every thing we can try, when it's our time to make the final journey, we cannot outrun fate.

Again, we have beliefs—some serve us, some don't; but we simply don't have enough information to state beliefs as irrefutable facts. Some of this conversation should be enjoyed as philosophical and spiritual discussions, like in the ancient bathhouses. What we do know is that we can exercise some control over what happens once we get here.

Until you take your last breath, you have options—about almost everything (always about the thoughts you think), including how you manage your health. You can choose mainstream (allopathic), holistic, or a combination. Your choices may be based on religious beliefs, social values, scientific knowledge, metaphysical beliefs, cultural beliefs, advice of professionals, as well as input from friends and family. You can choose to choose.

I truly feel that whatever the bodily condition, sweat therapy, when administered properly—and with very few exceptions as described in the previous chapter—should be an integral part of your detoxification and health improvement program. It should even be part of your dis-ease treatment program, should your body become too toxic for your eliminating channels. Only you can decide which route to take. I can only offer some knowledge based on my own observations and those of healing colleagues around the world with whom I have been fortunate and blessed to work with as one of the directors of the University of Natural Medicine.

The famous comedian and actor George Burns was once asked, "What is the key to long life?" He replied, "Don't stop breathing." It is not just important to breathe, but to breathe properly. Even pregnant women are taught to breathe a particular way in Lamaze training to assist the delivery process. Proper breathing can restore health. Three deep, deliberate breaths when you feel tense can do wonders. Proper breathing helps you create a highly-oxygenated environment and an alkaline pH (non-acidic) balance in your body. In addition, though discussed earlier, learn the art and science of proper fasting. Almost every serious health book has some recommendations on this topic. And find a way to sweat—a real sweat, and often.

We talked about standard drugs used by allopathic health care. These conventional therapies direct you to take as many highly-toxic sub-stances as you can handle. You've seen this cycle. It starts with one drug that is supposed to manage (not always touted as able to cure) an imbalance or disease. Then the side-effects start and another drug is prescribed to manage (not eliminate) that. Seventy-five percent of Americans over fifty are pharmaceutical "drug addicts." The American Medical Association admits that prescription drug side-effects are now the fourth leading cause of death in America. Many doctors even get cash bonuses when they prescribe drugs. This is, of course, done under the guise of "clinical research" being conducted within the framework of their practices.

Go into the home of an elderly person and find the tray on the kitchen counter with all the bottles of prescriptions they have to take on a daily basis. One woman saw that her elderly mother kept declining in spite of her many bottles of prescribed medications. She did something bold, though I'm not advocating this action—she flushed every pill down the toilet. Within a few days, her mother was once again alert and energetic.

Another example is a favorite treatment for a disease named myasthenia gravis. This disease is one where signals between nerve endings get confused. When chemicals are fired between the synapses, the nerve endings don't read them as signals to follow, but as ones that are attacking. The favorite treatment of this disease is to prescribe a pesticide to control symptoms and to remove the thymus gland—a gland critical to the immune system. These are drastic measures for a disease that has been successfully managed by just a couple of Chinese herbal protocols. Another example is the use of Coumadin, a blood thinner used to treat cardiovascular disease. This is actually warfarin sodium, known to many in its use as rat poison. Really, now, aren't there other choices?

It is sad to say, but true, that allopathic drugs, in general, add more poisons to an already overloaded system. As I said, people have a right to choose how they manage their health. Also sad is that many turn this management over to a doctor without ever getting any more involved than showing up for examinations, tests, and usually invasive, exploratory surgeries and at the pharmacy to fill prescriptions. This is like being in a fast-moving waterway in a boat with oars, but never picking them up to row. Some people just let the stream carry the boat, even if it's towards the edge of a waterfall or into rocks. My hope is that because you are reading this book, you've decided to row your own boat.

Onto the Next Level of Health Care

Are you now ready for the quantum leap? Extraordinary challenges demand implementing extraordinary measures. Oxygenation therapies are truly this next level.

Many persons in the U.S., including the famed diet guru, Dr. Robert Atkins, have been presented with their license to practice, then lost it and the freedom to use this therapy or advocate its use. *Ozone therapy*

(O₃) is the granddaddy of oxygenation therapies that's been legally, safely, and successfully used as the backbone of treatment for cancers, AIDS, and other life-threatening diseases in many other countries. Along with this is also *Hyperbaric Oxygen Therapy* (HBOT) and *Hydrogen Peroxide Therapy*. Different means of administering ozone exist. It can be administered directly into the vein as straight O₃. This has been touted by many international experts as the most potent and effective means and potential to cure life-threatening diseases. Ozone can also be mixed with removed blood and put back into the body (extra-corporeal blood therapy) or mixed with physiologically-compatible solutions such as saline. Another noted individual in the field, Ed McCabe, also known as "Mr. Oxygen," offers insight in case after case, where people were healed and disease eliminated from their body by using oxygen therapies as a cornerstone of treatment.

H.E. Sartori, M.D., Ph.D., another authority who is currently being persecuted and prosecuted (remember Linus Pauling?), has written the ultimate book on ozone therapy entitled, *"Ozone: the eternal purifier of the earth and cleanser of all living beings."* According to him, the direct intravenous route is the most effective means of eliminating disease and a powerful means to help prevent disease. Because of the very few deaths amongst the tens of thousands of persons treated—perhaps, due to the fact that something coincidental might have taken place within their bodies or the occasional inexperienced practitioner, this route is considered a dangerous one by the standard health care system. Sure, in the wrong hands, this can certainly be true—about any treatment modality. This is why training is so important. But, compare the numbers of people who've died from correct complementary care vs. totally standard (allopathic) care—or, mismanaged care in both fields. Dr. Sartori has documented scores of cases where people were rid of life-threatening diseases using his protocols in Sri Lanka. By creating a super-oxygenated body, this agent (oxygen), in combination with other lifestyle protocols (nutrition, sweat therapy, and mind-body medicine) fights disease most effectively.

An amazing technique that I have created, developed, and teach as part of my curriculum at the University of Natural Medicine and the World Organization of Natural Medicine is the use of vibrational frequency-enhanced ozone therapies injected into the specific acupuncture points in the body. This is a truly unique combination of millennia-old Chinese medicine with the ultra high-tech principles of the modern (not yet utilized by the allopathic) system of medicine. Since chi or life force energy, composed of electrolytes, lymphatic life-fluid, nutrients, blood cells, oxygen, and other bodily components travel through these channels, why not super-charged oxygen?! Deliver it so that it goes right to the end-target organ, where it is needed most! Other oxygenation therapies can be explored in my course under the same name on the website of the University of Natural Medicine (www.universitynaturalmedicine.com).

As a complement to ozone, I recommend that you explore U.V.B.— *ultra-violet blood purification therapy*. This technique draws blood, passes it through a small apparatus akin to a tanning salon effect, then is re-administered into the body. This apparatus contains a powerful ultra-violet light which negates and cleanses impurities, poisons, and biological organisms from the blood. Increments of 50-100cc are purified at a time. Instruments are continually being developed to combine the protocols described here.

Chelation therapy is a remarkable modality that should be strongly considered. Although different variations of this therapy exist, generally, a mixture of very large doses of Vitamin C, trace minerals, and EDTA (ethylenediaminetetraacetic acid) is slowly administered to the patient as an I.V. drip (intravenous). The blood vessels are stripped of disease-causing deposits and heavy metals. There are many examples of people who are ready to have heart by-pass surgery and other ailments, and, reportedly, have become completely well with this technique. You won't find this technique endorsed by the allopathic system, though. They denounce it as quackery, in spite of the results. They attack it vigorously. Why don't they give equal comment to some of the more "barbaric" treatments used in standard care throughout the ages?

These techniques I've just described should be done in conjunction with sweat therapy in order to increase the effectiveness and success of detoxification and re-balancing of overall health The next chapter delves briefly into sweat wisdom for those who engage in sweatier activities than most, whether occasionally or on a consistent basis. However, it contains valuable and potentially life-saving information for everyone.

Now, ENJOY great health!

"There's a lot of blood, sweat, and guts between dreams and success."
Paul Bryant

ATHLETES AND PERFORMERS
PROFESSIONAL AND WEEKEND WARRIORS:
Naturally-Occurring Sweat Therapy?

I decided to add this chapter to this book which is, after all, about sweat and the many benefits of sweat therapy. People in athletics or vigorous dance- or performance-related presentations must "know sweat," despite the fact they don't necessarily engage in these activities in order to get to a state of "no sweat." For them, it is a by-product of their chosen activity, but one which they must know well—not only for their performance, but for their health and, perhaps, survival. This is why I feel it is a "must read" section. As you'll see in the information included, some of it should be known by everyone, no matter their activity level.

This chapter is also important to me since I served as a physician for the U.S. Karate team in various international tournaments including the Karate Olympics in Manila, Philippines, under the directorship of my teacher and dear friend, former world champion, Terrence "Tokey" Hill. I have been personally engaged in athletics for a good portion of my life.

Most people involved in vigorous sweat-producing athletics or performance activities derive a natural sweat therapy in the course of doing what they do. If you are one of these, or even a weekend warrior type (or not), please read on. Professional dancers, boxers, runners, wrestlers and so forth, can sweat so much that their main problem is no longer elimination of wastes or stimulation of various body systems, but a condition known as *hyponatremia*.

This condition occurs when blood sodium concentration falls to an abnormally low level, promoting a rapid and dangerous swelling of the brain that can result in seizures, coma, and death. While this is a rare condition, it has resulted in deaths of marathon runners and military recruits. Though this condition results from prolonged exercise, believe it or not, it has the potential to occur when too much fluid is consumed while at rest. That's right. **You can literally drink yourself to death, and not at your local bar, but from over-consumption of good old water drunk while sitting in your favorite chair.**

Water intoxication, also known as *symptomatic hyponatremia*, is created when the body cannot excrete the consumed fluid rapidly enough to prevent intracellular swelling sufficient to produce neuropsyhological damage and, ultimately, death. In this condition, serum sodium levels fall to below 130- to 135-mmol/l (millimoles-per-liter).

Water is the main fluid which is needed by the body to support its life-sustaining functions. Water represents up to 73-percent of lean body mass. Body water is distributed between cells and in the plasma. At rest, approximately 30- to 35-percent of total body mass is intracellular fluid (in the cells), 20- to 25-percent interstitial fluid (between the cells), and 5-percent in plasma. During vigorous exercise, the elevation of extracellular tonicity results in water moving from the intracellular to extracellular (out of cell) spaces. From there, it can move out of the skin as sweat to keep the body from over-heating. The negative effect of all of this, of course, is potential loss of more water than is tolerable by the body.

By now, we all know that sweat is the obvious manner in which the body loses water. We also lose water via vapor through intense exhaling which takes place during vigorous athletics or activities. When we exercise, both routes are utilized fully and have a sound physiologic purpose. However, loss of too much water leads to yet another problem—*dehydration.* Water loss of even 1- to 2-percent, can stress the body's physiologic mechanisms and lessen one's ability for motor skills and physical activity. When we get to the 2- to 3-percent stage, this is like reaching the red line. After a 3-percent loss, physiologic functions which are further disrupted, cause an increased possibility in an athlete (or others) to develop exertional heat illness, i.e., heat exhaustion, heat cramps, or heat stroke. This level of dehydration is common in sports and can be seen after as little as one hour of vigorous exercise.

A rise in core temperature during exercise is a key physiologic finding in dehydration. For every 1-percent of body weight lost due to sweating, we see a core temperature rise of .15°C to .25°C. At very high (pre-dehydration) levels, the body tries to prevent catastrophe by diminishing the dilatation (expansion) of surface skin blood vessels so it can, therefore, sweat less. It is truly an amazing mechanism. Try to abuse it less.

The National Athletic Trainers' Association (NATA) has some sound recommendations for fluid replacement. Since this book is about therapeutic sweat therapy and not sports, I will not go into too many specific details. Remember, this book is to be a guide so you can Know Sweat—and, so you can know far more about sweat than you ever thought you needed to and why it's important that you do so.

Some guidelines established by NATA:

(Remember, though I use the word *exercise* to simplify, what follows applies to any extended high-level activity.)

•Consider the dynamics of the sport or activity, taking into account the rate at which the athlete or performer is sweating. Hydrate according to the allowable and practical confines of the activity, i.e., during breaks or time-outs, etc.

•Begin all exercise sessions well-hydrated. This includes ballet and dance regimens for performers, as well. As a rule, pre-exercise weight should be relatively consistent throughout exercise sessions. Body weight is dynamic. Check urine for color and match it against a chart as a good marker. Dark, of course, is concentrated. Very light means that there is much more water than dissolved particles. A rule of thumb might be (with the exception of how some supplements add color), when urine is clear or nearly clear, you're probably drinking enough water. Pre- and post-exercise weight (minus meals, defecation) should be fairly consistent.

•Consume 500-600ml (17-20fl.oz.) of water or a sports drink about 2-3 hours before exercising and about 300ml (7-10fl.oz.) of either of these fluids about 10-20 minutes before starting to exercise.

•Replace lost fluid during exercise whenever possible. Fluid replacement should approximate sweat and urine losses to maintain hydration at less than 2-percent of body weight reduction. This means that 200-300ml (7-10fl.oz.) should be consumed every 10-20 minutes. Once again, this should be in accordance with individual needs and based on the conditions and type of sport or other activity—not on published tables. Since there are many factors which affect gastric emptying and assimilation of water or fluids consumed during exercise, do not assume that in the heightened adrenaline-laden competitive state, it diffuses right out of the digestive tract to the tissues where it is most needed.

•Ensure return to physiologic function by correcting fluid loss during exercise by re-hydrating within two hours after exercise. This includes consuming not only water, but carbohydrates to replenish glycogen stores and electrolytes (electrically-charged minerals) to speed re-hydration. This is important because during intense sweating, electrolytes, sodium, potassium, chloride, and magnesium are lost from the body, along with water. This loss is greatest in beginners. As the training deepens, retention is more efficient. Under normal conditions, a regular diet will meet energy and nutrient needs. However, in vigorous exercise and demanding events which go on for hours, replacements will be needed.

•Persons supervising athletes should be able to recognize basic signs that dehydration may be taking place: Headache, weakness, thirst, irritability, confusion, cramps, chills, nausea, vomiting, head and neck heat sensations, and decrease in performance. When these symptoms take place, transportation to a medical facility where I.V. re-hydration is available is mandatory.

Going back to what was said earlier, heat dissipation takes place via radiation, convection (a form of conduction), and evaporation. Each of these factors come into play (exercise? play?!) in relation to the ambient temperature (environmental), relative humidity, and exercise or activity intensity. As we see a rise in ambient temperature, conduction and convection mechanisms decrease greatly, and radiation becomes virtually insignificant. Therefore, heat loss from evaporation becomes the main heat-dissipating mechanism for the exercising athlete or performer. While evaporation may account for more than 80-percent of heat loss in warm, humid conditions, it may result in as much as 98-percent of cooling in hot, dry conditions.

Since this book is about sweat, you know by now that the sweating response is critical to body-cooling when exercising in the heat or in a heated environment. Therefore, any factor that hinders evaporation, such as high humidity and dehydration, has negative effects on physiologic function and performance. In addition, over-heating can take place. Mechanisms which allow the body's ability to dissipate heat are hampered. Heat builds up with very little cooling taking place. When these two conditions come together, a potentially fatal condition called *heat stroke* can occur. Having similar symptoms to dehydration (nausea, dizziness, headache, confusion, mental disorientation, clumsiness, collapse), this can ruin your day! Take the precautions listed previously.

One more thing, "weight-loss clothing" that keeps sweat in, can help create this problem during vigorous exercise. The idea is to have "no sweat" (after you sweat) and not keep it in. You'll lose enough weight by sweating—trust me. If you own these types of clothing, keep them in the closet, not on your body.

Stay hydrated! If you want more detailed information in this area, read the article in the *Journal of Athletic Training* (2000) entitled, "National Athletic Trainers' Association Position Statement: Fluid Replacement for Athletes."

Well, I worked up a sweat just thinking about that one. I may stick to moderate sweating in exercise and use of the other techniques I gave you. Luckily, these situations rarely, if ever, develop during therapeutic sweating—unless you are a true masochist and wish to see the other side sooner than later.

Here are some frequently-asked questions on "sweat and the athlete."

How much sweat do we have to lose before we begin to see impaired body function and performance?
As stated before, it can be seen in as little as 1-percent dehydration—only 1.5 pounds of sweat loss for a 150-pound person to begin to see impaired function.

How much sweat can an athlete lose?
A "heavy sweater" in a challenging activity, can lose more than three quarts of sweat during each hour of activity. Therefore, the dehydration risk goes up very fast.

Why do we sweat when we exercise?
To maintain a safe body temperature.

As a person becomes more fit, does the mechanism of sweat change?
Yes. They sweat more and sooner since they sweat more efficiently, as well as over a greater surface area.

Why do we get thirsty from sweat-inducing physical activity?
Blood volume is reduced; thus, sodium concentration of blood is increased which stimulates the brain's thirst center.

Are men better sweaters than women?
No. There is no difference. Both exhibit a wide range of sweat parameters; but, there has not been any measurable gender difference.

Why is dehydration dangerous?
Because it strains the cardiovascular system more than any other system of the body. An overall decrease is seen in the blood volume due to fluid loss. The heart must then contract more frequently and force-

fully to maintain the same stroke volume. Maintaining a safe core temperature becomes difficult since blood circulation is hampered.

Are sports drinks good for athletes and high-activity performers?
Absolutely! They help replenish electrolytes such as potassium, sodium, and chloride. They provide necessary carbohydrates. They hydrate the body. I don't intend to make a sales pitch, but I personally take Gatorade® when I engage in a physically-taxing athletic activity.

Is there a correlation between age and how much a person sweats?
This may surprise many persons, but the answer is no. Sweat ability is related to fitness levels and acclimation to heat. The more physically fit, the easier and greater the sweat. So, to some of you older folks (I'm included here), Dr. Bill says, "Go for the gold!"

MY STORY:
Some Personal and Extraordinary Experiences

My journey has been anything but ordinary. My inquisitive mind and quest for adventure brought new levels of learning and experience all along the way—and still does. Some of these experiences caused me to break a sweat and break into a sweat, to say the least. Curiosity did, almost, kill this cat.

Every day that I served as an anesthesia resident at the urban trauma hospital where I interned, I saw the most extreme situations of the human condition. The local stations gave details about certain news events usually after I'd dealt with the results of these incidents as part of the team resuscitating and reviving the people involved. Often as I watched peoples' lives slip away, my mind was filled with What-ifs. Aside from my assistance in treating massive trauma of every type, I was part of the surgical team that worked on just about every condition. It often felt like being a part of a M.A.S.H. unit in a war-torn city. The area of this metropolis was such a zone.

I was doing this work while also having to run to OB-GYN in the wee hours of the morning to help deliver children to children who should have been playing with dolls rather than bringing babies into the world through their too-young bodies. My 36- to 48-hour shifts involved these deliveries plus the hair-raising emergency room scenarios—all which played out repeatedly during my shift. Some of this looked as though it could come right out of a Stephen King movie. I partook in many major invasive procedures, removal of organs, and other forms of bodily invasion and humiliation. The list of my experiences could go on ad nauseam.

As I put patients under anesthesia, I would wonder what happened to bring a person, usually born with healthy organs and spirit, to such a degenerated level of human condition. Poverty and lack of education were contributors, for sure. I felt that one person's suffering was transmitted to and directly or indirectly affected all humanity. The angry young child, deprived of all of the good things he feels he deserves as much as anyone, may very well turn out to be the criminal who feels it is his right to take things from you, often by force on some dark street. Something was wrong with the big picture. As I later went through different specialty areas of healing techniques, images from that time would haunt my thoughts. One particular thought was certain in my mind and changed the way I looked at health and health care forever. The thought was that many of these end-stage conditions I saw could have been prevented with the right knowledge, resources, detoxification, and commitment to know more. The adage, "An ounce of prevention is worth a pound of cure," definitely applies to health care. I came to the conclusion that toxicity, of any kind (physical, mental, emotional, social) causes disease in the body and in society.

After graduating from Queens College (Bachelor of Arts in Biology), I went to dental school. I was pre-med, and had to get the all-important pre-med approval from the Committee Chairman and Advisor at Queens College. There was something of a personality clash between us; so, "god" told me bluntly, "Akpinar, give it up. You'll never be a doctor!" But I wanted to be a doctor. I knew my purpose in this life was to heal. Didn't he realize that I'd healed animals as a kid? That I truly love helping others? He didn't approve of my B-level grade point average (gpa). For him, only a 4.0gpa indicated doctor potential. I believed dedication to healing was more important than a 4.0 in calculus, physics, and other non-relevant courses included in the medical training curriculum. I later saw, unfortunately, what some cut-throat pre-med students became...cut-throat doctors. This is why most of my friends are artists, musicians, and spiritually-oriented people. There are healers in their midst.

As I said previously, my own roots are in Turkey. I come from a lineage of doctors, famous journalists, Sufi masters, and the family historically responsible for taking the country out of the dark ages of ignorance and making it a Republic. I decided to re-visit my roots and pursue the next part of my studies abroad. To say this became an adventure is an understatement. I was accepted into dental school by way of a grueling examination. My decision at that time, was to finish dentistry, then medicine, then become a facial surgeon. This field held a kind of intrigue for me, I always loved aesthetics. People who have the astrological sign of Cancer in their make-up usually do.

While the first two years were relatively peaceful, the last two rocked my world and nearly brought it crashing down. A revolution engulfed the entire region. When I look back, I see that I always seemed to be in the wrong place at the wrong time. I was in the middle of one of the most publicized, violent political events which included cross-fires, bombings, and other incidents while waiting for a bus or a plane. Imagine how weird it was to see people drop to the ground as bullets ricocheted off the wall behind me. The sadly misguided persons who took it upon themselves to form "morality maintenance squads," would visit me and my friends to ensure that no morality-violating behavior was taking place on "their watch." Little did they understand that repressed sexuality equaled heightened potential for violence. Where the heck else would all the testosterone go? Such repression creates an environment that's like a pressure-cooker ready to explode. Judging from the history of the region, it quite often does. They apparently hadn't heard (or agreed with) the phrase, "Make love, not war."

I was an American living in Turkey, even though I was from there. I had to get accustomed to the water, food, and cultural traditions. The scars on my head and cracked skull are reminders of having fought off members of death squads who victimized potential targets, usually in the middle of the night, only to disappear as quickly as they appeared. My efforts to convince these individuals that I was a dental student and not involved in the revolution failed. Not wanting to be crippled for life like those they tormented around me, I once found myself in a situation where I had to execute a front snap-kick to the face of one of the leaders, followed by reverse punches and roundhouse kicks. That incident shaped my view of violence—how horrendous it truly is. This violent time of my life planted the seeds of my eventual gravitation to Buddhism and Taoism as philosophies and practices. My black-belt mastery of Tae Kwon Do, the Korean art of self-defense, allowed me to protect myself as I attempted to get on with my life, though a two-by-four did catch the back of my head when I missed a block. Nevertheless, they got the worst of it!

Amidst this chaos, I managed to travel through Europe and other Mid-Eastern countries and, unwittingly—as crazy luck or coincidence would have it, continue to find myself in other countries also in the middle of their revolutions! Yet, I managed to live through terrorism and watched helplessly as people all around me were taken away to be tortured—and worse. I nearly lost my own life on several occasions simply by standing my ground and not budging. In spite of this, I still got my dental and medical training—though I doubt the Chairman at

Queens College would have considered my accomplishments, in spite of the odds, as worthy as that 4.0 in calculus.

Ironically, when I was invited to give a lecture on alternative medicine many years later at my old college—a healing modality that was just beginning to raise a few eyebrows in the medical community—guess who I spotted in the crowd attentively listening to every word about this new medicine? I, of course, ended the lecture by indicating that a person in the audience had not considered me doctor material. Weird circle of life! And this is another reason we shouldn't judge anyone. Through all of this, I gained much experience and wisdom about life, something that would not have happened in the secure American medical school environment I had believed so critical to my future.

When I returned to the States, I began my residency at a New York hospital, followed by my residency at the hospital where this chapter began. If you're wondering why a dentist would go into general anesthesiology, I'll tell you something you may not be aware of (I wasn't aware of it): It was dentists who developed the art and science of anesthesiology and pain control. Dr. William Morton was originally a dentist and, like myself, went on to become a physician, as well. He successfully performed a painless tooth extraction using ether at Massachusetts General Hospital in Boston in 1846. Most people consider him to be the "inventor and revealer" of anesthesia.

An unorthodox, brilliant physician and anesthesiologist was in charge of my anesthesia residency program. He believed that dentists should study with physicians and participate in every medical procedure since most of us had great manual dexterity skills. Those of us who worked under him gained enormous proficiency and had a safety track record better than any group of physicians not in the program. Many of the dentists did as I did, and later became physicians.

The proficiency and safety track record mentioned in the above paragraph is, perhaps, due in some part, to the fact that medical equipment and supply people, non-doctors, of course, sold physicians the artificial hip and knee replacement devices and other gizmos, and to my fascination, diplomatically nudged the doctors aside and actually performed the critical parts of the surgeries, though assisted by the surgeons. They usually knew more about the procedures than the surgeons! I've seen many such procedures. A day in the life of an operating room.

Although advances have been made in the profession of anesthesiology, I personally witnessed two tragedies which still haunt me. On separate occasions, two patients from very poor neighborhoods—since urban trauma hospitals are usually located in such areas—were worked up by me the night before for benign elective procedures. Each was petrified about their procedure and considered cancelling their surgeries, altogether. I used all my skills to calm them down, believing that they would, indeed, be okay. Because of different medical mishaps while under anesthesia, which should have been prevented, both patients died. One involved the accidental disconnection of the breathing tube the automatic ventilator was hooked up to, by the resident I designated as in charge when I left for a break. He was too busy studying for his boards and turned the beeping alarm monitor off so as not to disturb his study time. Only when the surgeon doing the surgery asked why the patient's blood looked black, did they realize that the EKG screen had shown a flat-line for some time—with no alarm sounding, of course. The resident who worked with the other patient had initially placed the endo-tracheal tube in the esophagus instead of the larynx. The patient literally suffocated to death while under anesthesia, deprived of life-sustaining oxygen (going to his stomach instead of his lungs)—he couldn't "complain" because he was paralyzed anesthetically throughout the procedure.

I had to wheel each of them to the hospital morgue, passing the family being "consoled" by a senior staff member who was trying to explain that it was an "unforeseen" drug reaction. Complete B— S—! This same senior member also mentioned God and how the family should not be further tormented by defiling the body (read: autopsy) which, of course, would have revealed the true cause of death.

The phrase, "Doctors bury their mistakes," still has merit. The next morning at grand rounds, everyone was given a script and warned that if deviation from this script took place, it would be made certain that they never practiced anywhere in the U.S. Do you see why I'm a bit wary of the medical profession in spite of my own involvement with it?

A personal tragedy akin to this was the loss of my grandfather, Abdulhamit Yorga, due to a preventable medical error. Growing up in a family with limited financial means meant we had to take advantage of city hospitals and the worst chop-shop dental clinics—both meant for the poor. My beloved grandfather was a great intellect who survived not only Stalin but Hitler while living in war-torn Russia. He developed an infection due to a penetrating object and was given a treatment which he had an adverse reaction to, and had his life abruptly brought to an end by an arrogant physician. Whether this doctor was naturally arrogant or behaved that way because he viewed his "poorer" patients as less worthy is not something I determined. Rather than move my grandfather to the emergency room, they did the "next best thing," meaning medically and legally for themselves, and moved him into the elevator to die. This was the doctor's choice and directive—move my grandfather into a non-medical area so his death wouldn't go down as a medical error. I was a child then, but still vividly remember my mother weeping and pleading for this doctor to do something for her father.

Sadly, I saw several multiple-trauma cases handled the same way decades later during my residency. History and behaviors do, indeed, seem to repeat themselves. This was a catch-22 for me. If I spoke up, I'd be cast out and banned from becoming a doctor. I did this on several occasions in the residency and came within an inch of being thrown out. I later found out that a few senior residents used some "diplomacy" to handle the situation. I could only promise myself I would never treat any member of my human family with anything less than the dignity they deserved.

Living through such craziness in my training and, of course, previously in Turkey, I swore that if I ever got out of there alive, I would
1. Never sweat the small stuff in life ever again;
2. Live every day as if it could be my last; and
3. Stand up for injustice when I saw it, in every way possible—that when I saw it, I would do anything I could to counter it.

A quote by Dr. Martin Luther King, Jr., that resonates for me is, "Injustice anywhere is a threat to justice everywhere."

The combination of dental surgery and anesthesiology allowed me to help people in a big way. I eventually became director of pain management programs in two major New York City teaching hospitals working in anesthesiology, dental, maxillofacial, and surgical cases. For the next ten years, I primarily provided dental and reconstructive care to handicapped children and adults. This was fulfilling and made all my training and experiences worthwhile. I volunteered my services as a dentist and anesthesiologist at different charity organizations, dental clinics, etc. There was no way to place a price on the level of personal satisfaction and sense of purpose this experience provided to me. I know many in the medical field, enter it not for the sole (or soul) purpose of healing, but for monetary gain. Though I have benefitted financially, my dedication as a healer has always been foremost for me and I continue to give my all whether it's through compensated treatment or by volunteering my services. I don't say this tritely: I live to heal. This is my greatest satisfaction in life.

Always fascinated with Eastern medicine and philosophy, I went on to study acupuncture long before it became in vogue. To be honest, I was enthralled with this centuries-old system and the healing these methods achieved that I'd heard and read about. Initially, however, I remained a skeptic because of my hardcore medical training. I went on to train under some of the world's great masters including an internship with the Dalai Lama's personal physician while I was in Tibet many years ago, before it opened to the world. My training also took place in China, Taiwan, Europe, and other places. Though easy enough to become proficient and effective, it is nearly impossible to master acupuncture no matter how much training you get. It seems to be an art and science with no beginning and no end. Acupuncture combined with Western medicine can be especially effective. I became one of the first pioneers in facial and TMJ pain management (temporomandibular joint) to combine holistic with Western therapies in my field. Eventually, this was something I passed on to my students.

I wanted to learn more about the mind-body connection, so I studied biofeedback and hypnosis. Biofeedback is a high-tech measurement and treatment system based on the body's biophysical response to stress. This only whetted my appetite for even more. I went back to medical school at the age of 44 and graduated with my M.D. I had come full circle.

During all of this medical training, I continued in martial arts training, working for and getting three black-belts as I went along. Martial arts has parallels to the healing arts. Health is at the core of both. I've

studied over eight different styles of martial arts, but favor the
Chinese soft internal arts—particularly because I've sustained a few
injuries studying the hard ones. Martial arts have enormous healing
value for the mind, body, and spirit. I integrate these wisdoms into the
treatment of my patients.

So, I went from being a pain-management specialist to a detoxification advocate. I realized that most of my patients who came to me for
pain management had other underlying causes for pain than just the
trauma experienced from car accidents, falls, and so forth. A lot of
what I observed didn't add up. I began to make clinical correlations
from my large base of patients. Having first tried particular protocols
myself—a former smoker, junk-food eater, and weekend party-hearty
type—I began to recommend detoxification protocols to patients. And,
I observed how patients' health improved when I removed their toxic
amalgam fillings and replaced them with non-toxic ones.

But I wasn't finished with my studies. As far as I'm concerned, I never
will be. There is simply too much to explore and learn about healing
modalities. I studied with two great forensic masters, Cyril Wecht and
Henry Lee, as well as other noted authorities. These experts were, I
believe, involved in virtually every high-profile death investigation
including Marilyn Monroe, John and Robert Kennedy, Nicole Brown
Simpson, Jean Benet Ramsey, and so on. I was already Board Certified
in Forensic Dentistry, as well as Forensic Medicine (talk about a curiously morbid specialty!). These two men are medical and medical
legal heavy-weights who have forgotten more about pathology than
most of us can ever learn. I earned my designation as a Certified
Medical Investigator and combined this study with toxicology and
environmental medicine which gave me far greater insight into the
correlation between a toxic body and disease.

This was the beginning of a new path for me. My experiences are the reason I've embarked on a series of books known as Dr. Bill's Health and Wellness Series. I don't want this information that resulted from my experiences to be privileged. I want it to be widely-known so that individuals can make informed choices about their physical, mental, spiritual, and emotional health. Before I continue with the epilogue which is an interesting developmental phase of my life as I write this, I'd like to share some of my patients' stories with you.

Notable Case Histories* (and Notable Experiences!)

*ALL NAMES INCLUDED HERE, BUT ONE (USED WITH PERMISSION), HAVE BEEN CHANGED.

Dave

At 55, Dave came to me after seeing numerous doctors, with complaints of "just not feeling well." His physical exam and blood tests failed to reveal any immediate life-threatening situations. He was about 50 pounds overweight, had high blood pressure, the beginning of diabetes, and generalized pains. He did not sleep well and was usually tired during the day. And, he sweat constantly. His sweat had an ammonia-like quality to it which hit you as soon as he walked into the room.

I asked about his lifestyle and habits. He had the same malady most American men (and women) in his age group have: Tough job, mortgage issues, kids in school, no time for exercise, junk food on-the-go between meetings—you know the picture. I asked him what some might consider a strange question: Did he want to see his children complete college? Of course, he said yes. I told him I didn't have all of the answers, but could make some recommendations.

Before recommending any type of treatment, I implemented a mix of super green foods (chlorophyll, spirulina, and chlorella) to begin detoxification. I included vitamin therapy with 5,000 units of Vitamin C, 80 grams of B-complex, minerals, and a healthy dose of 300+ mg of Coenzyme Q-10. Within a few days, he seemed to come back to life. He modified his diet and added Omega 3 oils along with colonic cleansings. On his next visit, his "scent" did not precede him. Previously, my assistants had their hands on the air-purifier sprays the moment he left. His general energy, I will refer to as *shen*—spirit as called by the Chinese—was remarkably improved. His eyes were clear and he was beginning to grasp how important his health was to him. This was great, but the next step proved remarkable.

I got him to agree to engage in sweat-producing activity. He started exercising and using the sauna at his local gym. He literally sweated the poisons out of his body. When he first began his sweat therapy, he felt light-headed, dizzy, and nauseous—something many feel when they begin a detox program. The years of alcohol, medications, and other toxins were being cleansed from his body. Today, his energy and spirit are stronger than ever. His blood tests are great. Blood pressure is normal, diabetes gone, and he is 60 pounds lighter. Even his sex life improved. And why not? The quality of your sex life is an extension and mirror of your general health.

Expanded Comments
Many times, all that is needed for optimal health is to first, detoxify the body then second, detoxify the lifestyle. Work supplies many things to many people. Not all of us have the same requirements of a job. But neither should a job or a lifestyle (or a relationship) steal quality of life from us. If we truly feel stressed more than not, exhausted by life, or overall discontentment, this is a signal to us to look for a better way. To not do so, pretty much always leads to some kind of breakdown, whether in the body or the spirit.

Steve

Steve, 38-years old, was a young doctor who was on top of the world. As a child, he had severe scoliosis and was just a notch above being labeled disabled. Who helped him live a normal life was a highly-talented chiropractor. With this treatment, Steve went from cripple to normal in a short period of time. He made this chiropractor his role model and followed in his footsteps, becoming a chiropractor, himself. He simply revered this healer.

After graduating from chiropractic college, his mentor gave him his first job in one of his greatly-expanded practices in New Jersey. Under his mentor's supervision, Steve's early healing miracles, much like his own experience, multiplied all across that State. There was one problem: Some took on an "how dare he" attitude about a doctor expanding his healing services (called "over-utilization") into poor, Black, Hispanic, and other indigent communities and billing insurance companies for the services patients received which, of course, were allegedly not received or, even more incredibly, deemed not necessary by some clerk in an insurance company office trying to make a match by "analyzing data" and reporting it to higher-ups in the company. Politicians who promised "lower insurance rates," cited doctors as the villains; and in a campaign platform, systematically destroyed the lives of many.

Thus, started the investigation. Steve's mentor was systematically destroyed, as well as scores of young doctors working for him as they started out. So was Steve's health under this stress. He went from healthy, positive, and idealistic to depressed, physically depleted, and suicidal almost overnight. In short, he once again became a "cripple," if you will. He was diagnosed with Chronic Fatigue Syndrome. When I first met him, he looked like a scarecrow. His hands shook, he was terribly underweight, and couldn't concentrate. He had also been put on experimental drugs designed to supposedly save his immune system. Still, he was one of the lucky ones. Many of his colleagues just starting out, became the "lunch" of prosecutors looking to put notches in their belts and ensure votes. Little did I realize then that I would be subjected to the same experiences by the system five years later, initiated by the same entity, the most well-organized investigative insurance company around.

Since his prior doctors had placed him on a plethora of pharmaceutical drugs, my first approach with Steve was to get him into a spiritual detox program—not the usual approach of a physician. Megadoses of immune system-strengthening vitamins, minerals, and herbs were implemented. He began chelation and oxygenation therapies and I taught him qigong to help him begin to balance his inner, then outer, energy. His cold, clammy hands began to warm and dry. I introduced him to acupuncture, Chinese herbs, and Bach Flower Remedies. Once he was somewhat strengthened, I introduced him to sweat therapy.

The years of releasing vast quantities of adrenaline and noradrenaline, plus their build-up of toxic metabolic products in his system, had destroyed his adrenal glands and left his nervous, endocrine, and cardiovascular systems in shambles. His body was basically a toxic soup. All of this toxicity had combined with the toxic drugs he'd taken such as Interferon—taken, he thought, in order to stay sane through the methodical dismembering he underwent. It took many sessions before he was able to sweat. We approached his sweat therapies at a very low temperature, initially, because he would feel sick and on the verge of fainting.

He regained a semblance of normalcy; but, it remains difficult to regain full health as he is still under constant harassment and surveillance since he is on disability. But he is alive—a small miracle. He continues to follow his protocols in order to stay as healthy as possible under these extremely stressful conditions. Until they leave him alone, maintenance rather than full recovery, is all he can accomplish. Yet, sometimes the beauty of life is in the achievement of small miracles. One ripple at a time. One salvation at a time. Though Steve's story is not one of complete success, the fact that he is still alive and vastly improved indicates what certain protocols can accomplish even under extreme circumstances.

Expanded Comments
I could go into quite a bit of detail about the flaws in the insurance industry, but I won't—until I write the book, that is! I will tell you, however, that in the beginning of my own practice, I served as an insurance consultant in order to feed my family. I was unable to continue this for long though. Ironically, through a strange turn of events, I applied for a job in a mobile health clinic to take care of people's health needs in the ghetto, but dialed one of the phone number digits incorrectly. I wound up being given a job in a totally different entity as a "consultant," not knowing what it was at the time—which I accepted so my family could survive. This was very short-lived, indeed, because I found that my heart and mind could not align with being expected to deny over 80-percent of claims in order to save money for the insurance companies. The people I evaluated could have been my mother, father, siblings, or best friends. No, this did not last long, at all. According to my spiritual beliefs, they did hold these positions in my human family. I could not look in the mirror and be true to the healing oath I took and to my own soul. As stated in Maimonides' oath: "Let not the desire for wealth or benefit blind me from seeing the truth. Deem me worthy of seeing the sufferer who seeks my advice."

The straw that broke this (Turkish) camel's back was the morning I saw an ashen-grey near-corpse sitting in my waiting room. Not having looked at the appointment book yet, I asked him who he was and what

I could do for him. He said that because of his failing heart, he had at best, four to six months to live and was anxiously waiting (for some other poor soul to die) for a heart transplant. The immuno-suppresive drugs he was taking were killing him—and his teeth. His insurance company sent him to me to examine his teeth to determine if he needed dental work so he could eat and, therefore continue to live, while waiting for the new heart.

When he opened his mouth, I fought the urge to gasp. Whatever teeth he had left were infected, pus-laden, and loosened in the extreme. They were actually flopping around in his mouth as he gave me his medical history. A few implants to stabilize a denture would allow him the dignity of eating like the human being he was. I called the insurance company clerk who was handling his case and recommended they let him have this procedure done. Well, how dare I?! I was told the patient didn't need the implants, just a few dentures flopping about in his mouth would have to do—cost containment! I gave them my findings report.

At the time, I was still a consultant, but beginning my own practice and lived next door to my office. Bad move. I don't recommend it. Soon, the phone was ringing into the middle of the night! The clerks, in ascending order all the way up to the Vice President of the company, started pleading with me, demanding that I change my report. They asked why I wasn't being rational and seeing the reality. I told them my opinion was final. Some choice words, most too profane to include here, were exchanged on both sides. I lost track of this poor soul. They probably paid someone to write a more "rational" report.

Artie
A quiet, heavy-set meat-and-potatoes kind of man in his early fifties, had every indication that his health was not good. He'd worked in a

garage with massive amounts of chemical toxic pollutants for over twenty years, and I surmised he'd picked up enough airborne chemical and solvent carcinogenic exposure to cause serious problems. Sure enough, he developed lymphoma, a cancer of the lymph nodes.

Initially, he came to me with stress management issues exacerbated by an inability to sleep well, mild hypertension, and diabetes. We gave him a thorough checkup including a full array of blood tests. What was a surprise was his dark field microscopic evaluation. Fields of fungus, liver-stress indications, stacking and clumping of red blood cells (called *rouleau*), crystal formations, and most importantly, large clumps of mucous plugs were apparent. The latter concerned me more than the other findings. In virtually every case where these are found, cancer is soon to follow or is present, as in Artie's case.

His lifestyle, job, diet, and, unfortunately, his body stunk. A faint-to-moderate ammonia-like smell oozed from his pores in spite of frequent showers. His diet included way above the recommended daily protein limit. Junk food, during a 15-minute lunch break, was his lunch. Though not a smoker or drinker, everything else about his life was toxic. I implemented a detox program of green foods, green drinks, and a vitamin and mineral supplement plan. We modified his diet and he began to contemplate a career change.

Within three weeks, his blood profile changed dramatically. He had more energy, slept better, was more relaxed, and felt better in general. After two months, his blood looked virtually normal and he felt even more energetic. In case you're wondering, sweat therapy was included, which he did by using the health club's sauna three to four times a week. This detoxification process caused him to experience the effects of expelling huge amounts of toxins. In fact, at a certain point of therapy, his body was releasing the chemical pollutants causing the disease. He could not only smell them in his sweat, but taste them, as well! When treating a patient with cancer who has had chemotherapy, the body will expel the residual aspects of the chemotherapy lodged in the fat and other tissues. Patients often cite smelling and tasting these. This brings them back mentally and emotionally to the sad, scared, and depressed point in their lives, and we usually then deal with the spiritual component.

Artie took sick leave from work. His eyes cleared and his skin went from rough and coarse to smooth. He got his health and strength back and moved his family to Florida to start a different line of work and a renewed life.

Expanded Comments
Many people are unaware of daily dietary requirements. It is preferable that protein not exceed 30 grams per day. Ideally, a serving should be no larger than the size of your palm. Saturated fats should make up no more than 10-percent of total caloric intake per day. One thing you might want to research is the food pyramid presented to the general public. The original pyramid created was quite different from the one that emerged after the government and certain influential food conglomerates became involved with it. Conventional "then," is not what conventional is now, and certainly not what it will be tomorrow. As time goes by, the pyramid has been "tweaked" because enough knowledgeable members of the general public balked. But it still has not returned to the original recommendations. The high-protein diets, followed by the (simple) high-carbohydrate ones that emerged over the last several decades, have left in their wake, a large number of people with arthritic and diabetic conditions, and, certainly, more obesity than ever found in our history. Quite a score for those with financial interests in promoting certain foods and subsequent medical treatments. Briefly back to "conventional," there was a time when the pub-

lic was told that smoking cigarettes was good for health—that it calmed and relaxed the nerves—so was, therefore, beneficial. There are far better methods to achieve a relaxed state.

Jannee

An attractive 40-year old African American woman, a real head-turner, came to see me. She had much going for her and was also a party-hearty type. She partied until the first signs of trouble began to show. Still beautiful, I had to wonder what she had looked like before her problems began. Jannee had shared needles while experiencing the high of speed balls (mixture of speed and heroin) that had left her with HIV. The ugly Kaposi's sarcoma in her mouth was the initial sign of a problem. This was followed by shock, disbelief, devastation, weight loss, aches, pains, constant infections, insomnia, depression, and lack of will to live. Jannee had no energy left when she came to me. In fact, she came to me after being released from an AIDS treatment center so she could go to a hospice and die. I take them all in, these lost causes, a sign of my astrological predilections, if you wish, but definitely my dedication as a healer.

Her health insurance had run out and no one wanted to treat her. She'd been through all the AZT fixes, which like chemotherapy, tend to kill off healthy T cells. She'd also had protease inhibitors, intended to block enzymes needed for HIV replication known as the famous drug cocktail used to treat HIV. The side-effects of this cocktail include diarrhea, vomiting, fatigue, headaches, and fever. Other tests on Jannee showed additional catastrophic findings, though not surprising.

I had a straight-forward discussion with her, convinced her to stop smoking and give up the drugs she was still using in her effort to cope with her panic and depression. I knew we needed to immediately oxygenate her blood with super green foods, blue-green algae, multi-vitamins, Coenzyme Q-10, and a concoction of Chinese herbal teas to boost her liver and kidney chi functions. Ginseng was used, as well. She was given massive doses of Omega 3 oils, told to cut out all simple carbohydrates, fats, and eliminate caffeine and alcohol—her primary escape tonic. She actually listened.

Bach Flower Remedies (Rescue Remedy at the top of the list) were used to bring her devastated spiritual and emotional energies into balance. Homeopathic remedies were also prepared for her. One must attack the emotional component of the disease so that the patient doesn't have to revert to behavior that might, probably, bring it back. I gave her acupuncture three to four times a week. A course of oxygenation therapies was initiated and showed phenomenal results. She went to a local gym and used the steam room to raise her body temperature and sweat. She could not afford a far infrared sauna at the time, which is what I suggested. Remember, HIV is heat-sensitive and oxygen-sensitive. After 30 minutes, 40-percent of HIV inactivation in a 107.6°F bath has been documented. She also took a course of colonic hydrotherapy.

Within a matter of a month, we began to see a different person emerge. We considered it somewhat miraculous; but this is another situation allopathic health care would dismiss as anecdotal. After two months, her T cell and CD4 cell counts were at virtually normal levels. She gained back most of her weight and became the spunky, beautiful lady she once was. You would not recognize her as the same woman who came to my door.

When Jannee returned to the same treatment center that released her to die, the therapists' jaws dropped. They now beg to send people to our clinic. We never really know what the full plan for our life is; but with the right lifestyle changes, wisdom, courage, and faith (or belief), anything is possible.

Expanded Comments

Today, there are over 40 million people who are HIV positive or have AIDS. At least 25 million have died of the disease, and the numbers continue to grow. People routinely walk around like ticking time-bombs until some signs appear. A third of these do not even know they are infected. First signs are usually weight loss, diarrhea, the Kaposi's sarcoma Jannee had, fatigue, and just feeling run down.

AIDS is believed to be an umbrella for over 28 previously-known diseases and symptoms. Like syphilis, it may, in many ways, be the "great pretender." Of those who have died from this, 70-percent have been men, 30-percent women. In 2005, AIDS claimed approximately 3.3 million lives, of which 570,000 were children. Over 40,000 new HIV infections are reported in the U.S., alone, each year. HIV is set to infect 90 million people in Africa, causing 18 million children to be orphaned. And, unfortunately, over 25-percent of young Black men living in the ghetto, are believed to carry the HIV virus. It is estimated that 42-percent of HIV patients become resistant to the cocktail offered for treatment. I have witnessed cases where the HIV virus has been entirely removed from the body using the alternative treatments. There are cases in the literature.

Some early research was done regarding heat and the disease process. A paper was published in 1995, written by S. D. Owens and P. W. Gasper entitled, "Hyperthermic therapy for HIV infections," that highlights the anti-viral effects of fever therapy to support the, now clearly-demonstrated hypothesis that heat therapy may be beneficial as a therapeutic modality for persons affected. Quoted from the abstract, "Our hyperthermic hypothesis is based upon the mutant escape, quasispecies theory of HIV antigenic diversity. We propose that, if initiated during the asymptomatic stage of HIV infection, hyperthermia may prove to decrease the number of mutant HIV strains arising due to evolutionary pressures created by the patient's immune system, with a resultant prolongation of the asymptomatic period of infection. A review of the literature from three areas of investigation: the immune response to fever, heat as a tumor killing agent, and preliminary studies with fever and retroviral infections, strongly suggests that there is a good scientific basis for the use of hyperthermic therapy in a multimodal treatment approach to HIV infection." Further studies, though I feel not nearly enough, are being conducted to assess the inactivation potential of heat on the HIV virus. Expect some milestones on this from me!

Katy
This sweet, frail but spunky 32-year old mother of two beautiful girls, came to me to treat her pain that resulted from a motor vehicle accident that had occurred several months before I met her. Nothing she did made the pain go away. She was on her way to becoming another statistic in the category known as chronic pain patients. Her ailments included bad headaches, TMJ, neck and back pain—and, "By the way," she added—Multiple Sclerosis (MS). She mentioned it as though she understood there was nothing I could do about it, but should know she had it.

I started with the basics. Histamine is a compound the body releases during allergic reactions. This is formed from the essential amino acid, histidine. It results in various bodily responses, mainly dilation of blood vessels and contraction of smooth muscles. These responses, in some cases, have been reported to relieve MS symptoms. Acupuncture, when used vigorously, causes a histamine release, among other benefits. So does bee-sting therapy. I began Katy on a regimen of acupuncture two to four times a week, with vigorous needling. We also used auriculotherapy, otherwise known as the art and science of ear acupuncture. I referred her to a friend of mine who lovingly calls his bee hives his Bee Hyatt Regency. He gets and holds one of his buzzing buddies with tweezers and, based on the desired effect, holds the bee over an acupuncture point where the stinger is brought into contact with the skin. Depending on the desired effect and the tolerance of the patient, the stinger is left embedded in the skin for a desired length of time. As a result of this treatment, not only did Katy's headaches and TMJ begin to disappear, I was elated to see a totally different, happier person emerge over several weeks. I also recommended she remove all of her dental amalgam fillings.

She diligently did the set of qigong exercises I gave to her. Her coordination began to improve. I consulted with my dear friends and fellow members at the University of Natural Medicine, Drs. Larry Milam, Mark Smith, and James Zhou (mentioned earlier), about a specific nutritional protocol for her. It included high doses from the B-vitamin family, which has a strong effect on the nervous system. We increased her calcium intake and magnesium levels. These improved her muscle and nerve function. We included a heaping regimen of green-food formulas, Coenzyme Q-10, Omega 3 oils, and enzyme therapy. Her circulation was boosted by far infrared sauna sweat therapies.

After several months, her improvement was remarkable. A note of caution: People with MS must be cautious in using high levels of heat, initially. It is important to work up to a comfortable level of tolerance over time. But this is one of the benefits of far infrared heat therapy. In conjunction with all described above, Katy also did hyperbaric oxygen therapy (HBOT) and ozone therapy. Again, her improvement was remarkable. One has to wonder what her condition would be at this time had she never decided to attempt something different and just accept her fate.

Although I lost touch with her once she'd improved, I have been blessed to work with some great doctors at a state-of-the-art international healing clinic in the Bahamas and with others around the world. At these sites, we have developed protocols to not only detox, but for the successful treatment of some of the diseases labeled as incurable by the medical establishment.

Expanded Comments
Allopathic medicine has indoctrinated the belief in many, that there is nothing to be done about certain medical conditions other than treat the symptoms as best they can. Pain management is something insurance companies don't like because it messes with their cost-containment factor. And, unfortunately, by the time an MS diagnosis is made, the damage has already been done. Patients are convinced that the only results they can expect is relief from symptoms—no cure. Palliative care vs. patient care.

Multiple Sclerosis is more a curse than a killer. At least 350,000 Americans are afflicted. It is considered one of allopathic medicine's least understood diseases. Conventional medicine offers no cure for it. First diagnosed in 1849, it typically affects people between the ages of 20 and 40, and women twice as often as men. The layer of insulation (called myelin) which is responsible for the actual propagation of impulses and surrounds nerve fibers, develops patches of demyelination (loss of the myelin sheath or covering of the nerve). A possible explanation is that it is an immune system attack on the nerve sheath. My dear colleagues in Freeport, Bahamas, have an excellent track record of treating this and other diseases with Immunokine, a formulation made from diluted Thai cobra venom.

When the multiple nerve sheaths are lost, scarring or hardening occurs—called sclerosis. Nerve transmission and propagation of

impulses such as your brain telling your hand to lift, become disrupted. Increased fatigue, balance problems as a result of less-coordinated
muscle movements, and paralysis occur as the disease advances.
There is an increase in sensitivity to heat and cold, with heat reported to make symptoms worse in about 60-percent of MS sufferers—the
primary reason I was very careful about using and monitoring the far
infrared heat therapy in Katy's treatment.

Joe's Father

Joe's father was carried into my office. His legs were essentially useless, lifeless, purple-colored, pus-containing trunks as hard as the
wood his son, Joe, used in his carpentry trade. The man's legs were
just a hair away from amputation. He was 65, suffering, and appeared
to be at the end-point of his life after years of severe congestive heart
failure, a disease which, as noted before, carries a prognosis as grave
as cancer. He was brilliant, but difficult, and fought with his stoic wife
from the time they entered my office until the time they left.

His heart was failing. The backlog of fluids in his lungs was so
advanced he could not finish a sentence without coughing. He was
like a three-pack-a-day smoker, though he didn't smoke. His failing
heart had not only congested his lungs, but had backed up the fluids
into his lower extremities. The circulation was virtually destroyed in
them. He was way past the pitting edema stage where you push into
the flesh and an indentation or pit remains for a considerable time.
His toenails were full of fungus due to the lack of circulation. He'd
been in and out of hospitals for ten years receiving only palliative
(pain-relieving) assistance. The diuretics he was taking were deplet-
ing his potassium levels and doing nothing beneficial.

First used, was electromagnetic therapy in the form of treatment
known as diapulse, administered to the lower extremities in an

attempt to improve circulation. A radical combination of oxygenation therapies and ozone were applied to acupuncture points of his lower extremities. Acupuncture was also used to improve his chi flow. I have seen many of these types of situations where the extremities are so far gone that when the acupuncture needle penetrates the skin, it makes a popping sound followed by lymph fluid oozing out.

Natural diuretics replaced the conventional ones he could no longer tolerate and, eventually, we weaned him off the toxic drugs which threatened to kill him if the CHF, itself, didn't. We continued the oxygen therapies, changed his diet, added massive doses of healing and cleansing herbs, and introduced sweat therapy using the FIR sauna— the only one that should be used for this type of condition.

Miracles? His cough and wheezing stopped. He no longer needed to be carried, and used a cane to walk. The only thing I couldn't repair was his penchant for fighting with his wife. That was beyond my purview. Maybe I'll wear that hat in my next life.

Expanded Comments
Yet, again, we see in this instance, a person who, by virtue of all that was malfunctioning in his body, would have died prematurely had he not sought complementary treatment. Not only that, but the level of suffering he endured every moment of his life was relieved with these "non-standard" methods. Unnecessary suffering is one of the most tragic side-effects of the allopathic health care system.

Marcia
Slightly obese, smoked half a pack of cigarettes a day, no obvious health problems, and a relatively young age—41. Yet, Marcia had an annoying problem of coldness in her hands and feet. Let me rephrase that: Not annoying, incapacitating. Doctor after doctor told her she

had Raynaud's Disease—basically, cold extremity disease. It is characterized by constrictions; spasms of the smaller vascular system components; and affects the nose, tongue, and feet. This condition is one where symptoms initially occur in response to cold or emotionally upsetting situations. Fingers become bluish or reddish and blood supply to these areas is compromised.

I advised Marcia to begin either qigong or heated yoga (described earlier), or at the bare minimum, a sauna to induce sweating and get her chi flowing. I advised her to either cut down or quit smoking. Her other habits weren't too bad, but I wanted to see her level of initial compliance before we really got going. She chose heated yoga. We added nutritional support. Within a matter of weeks, her circulation improved and instead of suffering with Raynaud's Disease, she became a yoga instructor and now teaches others how to get well. Although I have a long way to go before I become a Buddha, I love helping people change their lives for the better!

Expanded Comments
Raynaud's Disease is more commonly found in young women. When it is a result of other health problems, it is called "Raynaud's phenomenon." This is one of those idiopathic terms—meaning it has no known cause. This usually translates into, "Since we don't know the cause, we don't know the cure." And, another palliative medication gets created and sold.

Gloria
Beautiful, loving, artistic, considerate, intelligent, clairvoyant—a typical Dr. Bill patient as my colleagues affectionately call these spiritual "New Age" types who always gravitate to me—and a 42-year-old corporate executive, when she came to me. Gloria lived with excruciating pain in her head and joints, dizziness, double vision, fatigue, TMJ, and pain in just about every part of the body you can think of.

Two events seemed to have a role in her condition. First, she was only several blocks from the Twin Towers when they were tragically brought down on September 11, 2001. She got a toxic dose of burning metal, fuel, human debris, and every other horror imaginable in her attempt to escape. Another was her medical history. She'd had major dental work done to begin to remove the amalgams and other metallic alloys that had been used in her mouth. We looked at her lab tests and did a live blood cell analysis on her. Her immune system was almost non-existent. The lymphocytes, neutrophils, and other white blood cells were so sluggish it was difficult to even recognize them as cells. Their numbers were also greatly diminished. There was evidence of liver stress, an indication of a highly-toxic liver overloaded with pollutants, as well as other toxins. She was always in pain and couldn't concentrate and, additionally, experienced periods of confusion.

We started chelation therapy, massive doses of antioxidants including Vitamin C, green foods and drinks, alpha lipoic acid, carnosine, carnotine, enzyme therapy, Chinese herbal teas, and oxygenation therapy. She wasted no time in having her dental work cleaned up and bought a far infrared sauna. She was determined to sweat the poisons out of her body. It was slow and tedious. Initially, the detoxification process exacerbated symptoms and caused her to feel worse. I described this somewhat earlier, but we call this the *healing crisis*. As I mentioned before, this results from toxins being released from storage in the fat cells into the body. She persevered through the good and bad days.

Her ashen-gray skin became rosy. Her nail beds began to show rebound blood circulation. The dark circles under her eyes began to disappear and her blood profiles improved. Quality of life has since returned to a remarkable and vibrant woman.

Expanded Comments

Many people who decide to detoxify their body are unprepared for the healing crisis I've described in this book. They almost want to stop, and some do, in order to return to a more "normal" way of feeling—akin to what they felt before, even if it wasn't all that good. It is important to realize that this healing crisis is temporary. It will pass. And how it manifests is different for each individual. You don't need to prepare for the worst, just be aware. If you feel unsure about this, seek out a qualified health care provider to make recommendations and guide you through this process. The morning will come when you awaken and realize you feel more rested and more even in your energy than you have in a long time.

Some are under a misconception about energy levels. Energy is meant to be evenly distributed throughout the day and only rise when absolutely necessary. Running on high can be just as detrimental as running on low. Generally, people who seek to detoxify are aware of the low energy level they feel. Don't look for or anticipate a high as your normal level, aim for even. As the Chinese say, moderation is the best way.

James and Marie

I'm not a fertility specialist, but these close friends of mine wanted to conceive a child and simply could not get pregnant. I knew their medical history: No drugs, smoking, hard drinking. Their only addiction was a love of Harley Davidson motorcycle riding—one I joined them in often with my own "FXR Low-rider model." This was cleverly removed from me by one of Dad's friends who, also cleverly (to protect me from becoming road-kill, I guess) claimed that he would fix a small problem free of charge. Whoopee. I'm still waiting for it to be fixed and returned to me—10 years later!—as I write this.

Anyway, I took up another thrill—professional drag racing—to supplement my need for endorphins at that time, with an alcohol-burning speed slingshot called a "rail"—the wickedest, fastest drag racer imaginable. Zero-to-sixty in one second—like going through the time tunnel! The only difference here is that if and, eventually, when you crash and burn, the flame is white hot and clear. Your fireproof suit is only good for about 15-30 seconds, at best. Your swift removal from the wreck is imperative in a fire of 2,000C+ —much hotter than a sauna!

Back to James and Marie. Sometimes the cause of apparent infertility is stress. This can become a vicious cycle for a couple since the more they try to cope with the stress of trying to conceive, the more stressed they get. I regulated Marie's nutrition and recommended she change her numerous amalgam fillings for non-toxic ones, taught her meditation and relaxation techniques including qigong, gave her Bach Flower Remedies and Chinese kidney chi-enhancing formulas, and put her on a detox protocol. Based on what I now know, every woman should engage in a two- to three-month detox before even thinking about getting pregnant. Same goes for the man whose sperm cells can be affected by his own toxicity. I used acupuncture treatments on the spirit, conception, and governing-vessel points, and kidney and bladder points (responsible for reproduction chi). Ironically, Marie decided to do Native American sweat therapies on her own—common with us Harley types. She beat me to the punch on this one! Three months later, Marie was pregnant—with twins—though, sadly, one died in utero. They cherish their beautiful daughter.

How many couples spend fortunes at fertility clinics, and years of frustration and stress, when there may be a simpler way? Not only that, my friends cleaned up their bodies which also gave their daughter a good start, right at conception.

Expanded Comments

When a couple has trouble conceiving, the first thing they usually do is have thorough medical tests to rule out specific problems. If they are found clear of anything that would prohibit conception, what remains is stress and toxicity—though the latter is probably not something the allopathic system would consider. Toxicity not only impairs bodily functions, but is believed to impair fertilization. A toxic environment, external and internal, is even being considered (by some) as possibly responsible for the surge in postpartum problems found in unprecedented levels today.

Sam

I first met Sam when he was a salesman—a witty, charming, hilarious human being with heart like no other. He sold me my first car, a Mazda RX-7. I had earmarked just enough in my budget (my very first paycheck was the down-payment) to buy the lowest priced, stripped-down version; but after talking with Sam, I was convinced I needed the super-stock, top-of-the-line racing version to celebrate getting my license to practice. He probably guessed that I had a heavy foot and a need for speed. My next car, the Porsche 911 Carrera, was one he helped me lease and came within a millionth of costing me my license to speed. It was quite a rush, one I now miss from time-to-time since I currently drive a more conservative, yet still fast, car. We immediately became more like brothers than just friends.

Sam's problem was obesity. We shared many interests and had many good times; but Sam had serious self-esteem issues and like many, used work to escape looking at his issues and resolving them. He had high blood pressure, diabetes, and heart disease. Sam was not moderately obese, he was overweight by about 200 pounds.

I began with acupuncture, focusing on the ear which is very effective against addictions—including to food. He went on a detox protocol with heavy supplementation of vitamin cocktails that included chromium to regulate insulin, stabilize blood-sugar levels, and prevent the build-up of fats. We used natural iodine found in kelp and trace elements to regulate his basal metabolic rate. He did colonic cleansings, saunas, and exercise. He lost over 150 pounds.

Though his life seemed to change dramatically for the better, something snapped, though he wouldn't confide what it was to me. I said we were like brothers, but Sam always kept a part of himself closed off. Sadly, we lost touch for various reasons, including a heavy travel schedule on my part. I later learned he had met with a psychologist who convinced him to enter a rehab program once he found out that Sam had a great insurance plan. This treatment brought heavy therapy, heavy drugs, and a heavy shock to his system. I returned from a trip to learn Sam had died. No explanations, no autopsy, no excuses. I delivered his eulogy. I truly felt the loss of my dear brother.

This was one of many defining moments that impacted my attitude towards the healing profession. I never learned what happened to cause his death. The system made sure that information was buried, like Sam, never to be fully known. During a period of grief, people are often so traumatized, they don't want any further pain—something an autopsy often elicits. It has been said sarcastically, as I did earlier, that sometimes, "Doctors bury their mistakes."

Expanded Comments

I mentioned previously that obesity is more than just about food consumption. Though high toxicity also contributes to weight-loss complications and the way people who are obese generally feel healthwise, emotional complications always exist—whether they created the tendency for obesity or are a result of them. God only knows what fragile part of the psyche was damaged at a tender age to induce nurturing through massive food engorging later in life. If obesity is not properly dealt with, it can result in tissue, organ, and system damage, as well as high blood pressure, diabetes, heart disease, and certain cancers—to name a few.

Up to 40-percent of people in the U.S. attempt to lose weight at any given time. It is not easy since there are many factors affecting the situation above and beyond our eating. An underactive thyroid, pancreatic dysfunction, poorly-functioning liver, and sluggish digestive system are big culprits. So is toxicity—not only of the body, but of the mind and spirit, as well. Many usually engage in the various big-business treatments of diet, exercise, supplements, psychological counseling, and medication.

It is an amazing, ironic planet we live on. Simultaneous to people struggling with obesity, many parts of the world struggle with starvation. The World Health Organization estimates that over 300 million adults, worldwide, are obese. A good deal of them live in the U.S.— more than half that number if we rely on statistics. Every year, 80 million Americans go on diets. Within 5 years, 95-percent of them gain back not only what they lost, but usually more. Fad diets never produce long-term results. Genetics do play a role, as do dietary lifestyle habits. Eating patterns eventually create a "set point" which the body tries to maintain. Once fat cells expand in number, they do not shrink.

Other causes of obesity include food allergies (you'd be amazed at how many are allergic or sensitive to dairy and processed flour), nutritional deficiencies, sluggish metabolism characterized by low basal metabolic rate (BMR), hypothyroid, insulin imbalance, and lack of exercise (a simple and often ignored path to wellness). According to the Center for Disease Control, a quarter of the population is sedentary, while over 50-percent are inadequately active.

Another culprit is a toxic liver. A liver loaded with toxins results in a build-up of fat, usually formed as "lymph fat." A congested, toxin-laden colon also creates this as the absorption of nutrients and removal of toxic waste is impaired.

Eating is pleasurable, for sure. Eating certain foods momentarily eases certain stress levels. Some cause a release of endorphins, the brain's "feel good" chemical, and natural pain relievers like serotonin which is a potent mood regulator. But eventually, the pleasure found in this over-consumption turns to pain. Food is also legal. No one will give you a ticket or prosecute you for over-eating. There is no law (yet) for possession of chips or chocolate. However, at the time of this writing, New York City is the first to ban trans fats from being used by any business that provides food for public consumption. Feelings are split between approval of a healthful "law" and disapproval of enforcing legislation about what people can eat.

Documentaries and news segments have demonstrated how obese people and those who donned suits and prosthetics to appear obese are treated in society. Though there are some cultures on the planet that place a high value on women with extra poundage, America is definitely not one of them. In fact, it is quite the opposite here, causing a disruption in self-esteem of normal, healthy women who would have to forgo eating, nearly completely, in order to attain and maintain the clothes-hanger bodies models and actresses are encouraged to have so that garments hang on them a certain way.

Media, fashion, and the entertainment industry have a tendency to convince women and men there are limitations as to how a successful, happy person should appear. I'd like to say they should appear, be, and feel fulfilled and healthy.

Sue

Sue was a beautiful, talented, thin, wiry 35-year old lawyer who loved to talk as long as anyone would listen. Her problem was consistent sinus infections, sore throats, and asthma. Her medical history wasn't peculiar, but her lifestyle was the complete opposite of a healthy one. Let's just say it involved junk food eaten on-the-go, five or more cups of coffee every day, moderate amounts of alcohol, little sleep, and tons of stress. In addition, there must have been the added stress of unspoken or repressed issues with her family (as many of us have), as well as the stress of performing as a lawyer where judges and attorneys continuously interrupt statements. All of this led me to consider how this affected her throat chakra (more about this in *Expanded Comments*).

Feeling compressed time-wise, she agreed to follow some of my suggestions such as to create a steam-bath for her sinuses by heating a pan of water, turning off the heat before placing her face over the pan (a must-do), and adding menthol to the water. She had immediate and excellent results. She did begin to use regular sauna treatments and, remarkably, considered a major lifestyle change—something I wasn't sure she would even contemplate. Sue adopted a nutritional regimen which cut down on mucous-forming foods, and made every effort to eat her last meal earlier in the evening. She followed the meditation exercises I recommended, though wasn't quite ready for my recommendation to use crystal healing to cleanse her chakras.

Expanded Comments

I have observed that certain areas of employment such as law enforcement, government, investigative, and prosecution cause people to live in a primarily negative energy. The work they engage in causes them to deal with aspects of society most of us usually don't have to give more than a passing thought to in our day-to-day lives. The chakra systems of the negative people they have to be involved with through tracking, apprehending, and punishing, and their own energetic chakra systems, seem to form a very unhealthy bioenergetic bond or connection. They often end up suffering from the same maladies of the people they deal with—a root- and survival-chakra syndrome. While something has to be done to keep people who choose criminal activity at bay, there are spiritual exercises that those in these professions should do to maintain their health and balance. Along with this, is the usual poor nutrition and eating habits, caffeine or other stimulant consumption, irregular hours, adrenaline surges, lack of adequate sleep and exercise—all contributing to a highly toxic physical and emotional environment.

These types of jobs also involve the throat chakra. For those not familiar with this, let me briefly explain that it is believed there are seven major body chakras, or "energy wheels," which correspond to areas of large conglomerations or plexi of nerves. They emit internal energy and receive what is termed universal energy. The throat chakra is often seen, bioenergetically, as the link between thought and action. It is the vehicle of expression. When the throat chakra is repressed, not only does energy become depleted, others often lose their desire to listen to the person when they speak. When this chakra is in a state of imbalance, the thyroid and parathyroid glands are affected. Every chakra system is associated with various organ and endocrine systems. All facets of body metabolism, including bone and muscle metabolism, become affected.

As in Sue's case, it isn't a surprise to find the sinuses affected, as well. There are four sinus cavities in the head. Inflamation can be caused by an infection and can involve a build-up of fluid in the sinus cavity. Thirty million people suffer from this, which translates into a six-billion-dollar-a-year industry. Prescribed and over-the-counter remedies never cure this, they simply treat the symptoms. Sinus problems and asthma are frequently found together. Mucous-forming foods such as dairy products and processed sugar and flour are often the culprits.

I mentioned food allergies earlier. Many are not aware that they are lactose-intolerant or allergic to anything made from antibiotic- and toxin-laden cow's milk.* This mucous forms a readily-available substrate for bacteria and viruses to hide, grow, and release their toxic metabolic products. Exposure to pollutants, overuse of antibiotics, poor work or home environmental conditions, bad air quality, tobacco and other smoke, dry air, and even the common cold can precipitate and exacerbate both conditions.

The many cases I have treated, revealed a common thread: Most have moderate to advanced levels of emotional stress. People who suffer from chronic sinusitis are often high achievers. They have a low tolerance for making mistakes and are quite hard on themselves. They seem to have a low tolerance for being human! These types would definitely benefit if they opened themselves to meditation and a more spiritual or metaphysical approach to life. Also, acupuncture—I have not had one person with these conditions fail to respond to this treatment.

*Many allergic to cow's milk have no problem with goat's milk or cheese products made from it. And, somewhat humorously, because of their placement in the dairy section of grocery stores, there are those who when advised to stop eating dairy, stop eating eggs!

Raul

When I met Raul, he was a 53-year old shaman from Central America, and we became fast and close friends. He was adept in the practice of shamanism and sweat-healing ceremonies. In his native country, it is common to add peyote, a cactus extract, to take the shaman and participant(s) to higher levels of conscious awareness.

His story is one of self-healing where I was a witness rather than a facilitator. A childhood of sexual abuse by a relative, and its effects, travels as a dark-shadowed companion throughout his life. He dealt with the issues of sexual abuse constructively, not only through his own sweat therapies, but through his activities as a leader in media film, mostly through documentaries on Native Americans expanded to include victims of sexual abuse, with a focus on children exposed to this. His films offer closure to participants and result in the seeds of understanding growing into compassion, forgiveness, and release. Though difficult for some to see as such, according to some karmic-based belief systems, personal challenges, especially when some form of pain and suffering are involved, are "gifts" the universal consciousness gives to us as opportunities to evolve to a higher spiritual and, even, more humanitarian level of consciousness.

I joined him in one of his sweat-healing ceremonies where he shared his story to the circle of individuals present, who were also there to seek clarity, hope, and closure. In this particular circle, was a successful singer who'd suddenly and inexplicably lost her voice; a person with chronic pain that did not respond to the different therapies tried; some with deep psychological scars; and, those looking for a connection to the divine. As the heat became intense and nearly intolerable, Raul chanted, sang, and prayed in his native dialect. Each of us took our turn to tell our stories. I witnessed amazing healings as a result. I said the effects of Raul's experiences walk like a shadow with him, but because of what he does and who he is, it is only a shadow—not a form that impacts his life in any way other than helping others.

The one extraordinary and distinguishing component of a shaman-led sweat ceremony or spiritually-based communal sweat is that there is a very strong component—prayer. Shamans are among the most advanced and attuned medical practitioners I have met in life. Through dedicated spiritual and personal sacrifice and development, they are able to harness and channel the beneficial vibrational universal energy through prayer. Quite simply, during a sweat ceremony, they pray for and heal the afflicted. The concentrated, pure vibrational energy they direct out affects the vibratory frequency of the most abundant fluid in the human body—water—and changes its quantum field wave frequencies to a much higher, better, and healthier (disease-free) frequency range. The heat used in the ceremony, expands the now-energized body fluids, and they permeate the body with new, charged life-giving energy. In this manner, the negative vibrational frequencies, mostly of bad or negative emotions, become refracted with love and compassion. The disease-causing wavelengths dissipate. Makes a person consider this as partial reason why certain cultural rituals such as communal bathing and sweats have endured for centuries. If this seems unlikely, recall Dr. Emoto's results of thoughts on water.

Expanded Comments

Raul is a man who does sweat therapy on virtually a daily basis. Though 53 when I met him, his skin looked half his chronological age. No wrinkles, crow's feet, lines—just smooth, baby-like texture. As a doctor, I don't feel it is presumptuous to assume his internal organs parallel his external and largest one.

Engaging in regular sweat therapy may require some time and energy, but look at the savings in costly creams and products that are not long-lasting, not to mention the expensive and dangerous cosmetic surgeries and injections that often result in an unnatural result. And, the other internal benefits are well worth the effort.

Mary

Fibromyalgia struck this 65-year old sweetheart, putting her in a wheelchair and unable to talk. Her body was so tender, you could hardly touch it to examine, let alone treat, her. She hurt everywhere, felt terrible all of the time, was fatigued, anxious, depressed, irritable, dizzy, allergic, and hardly slept. Not a good combination.

It is difficult to pinpoint the cause of this affliction; yet, I believed that an emotionally traumatic event in her life may have been involved or at the root of this. There were the expected dark circles under her eyes, her adrenal glands were wiped out, life chi was blocked. She couldn't talk, but she could make sounds. I gave her some chanting mantras and urged her to chant certain sounds. There are six healing sounds that when chanted, the vibrational frequency or resonance, vibrates internal organs and opens blockages. I applied medical qigong, used acupuncture to open energy blockages, and began her on Bach Flower Remedies—with, of course, Rescue Remedy at the top of the list. Chinese liver (to dissipate anger), kidney (to control fear which usually always manifests as anger), and ginseng-based teas were used. Friends of mine who are chiropractors and massage therapists volunteered their time to help her get well. Green foods were used to detoxify her liver channel and open her energy flow. I wanted to purge the toxic gunk from her energy meridians, so arranged to have her lowered into a hot bath, like a full-body Sitz bath, so she could sweat.

Mary is still in a wheelchair, but about a thousand times more functional than she was. She continues to work on her healing. It would not surprise me if one day, this remarkable woman walks again.

Extended Comments
Fibromyalgia, by definition, has been traditionally categorized as tenderness in 13 areas. According to the American College of Rheumatology, there must be widespread pain for anywhere from 3 to 11 months in the 13 painful, tender muscle sites. I find it amazing at how they need to categorize human conditions in order to grasp them as real.

People afflicted hurt everywhere, feel fatigued and, overall, just plain crappy. This malady presents a Chronic Fatigue Syndrome-like effect, with pain as the primary symptom. It is estimated that approximately 3-6 million Americans suffer with it, with 86-percent of those afflicted being women between the ages of 34 to 56. As many as a quarter of these are on some form of disability because of the impact on their lives.

Among factors cited for fibromyalgia are viral or bacterial infections, trauma from an assault or accident, psychological trauma, long-term stress, heavy-metal poisoning—including amalgam fillings, external poisoning from environmental and chemical factors, Influenza A... The list keeps going. Fibromyalgia patients also show two to three times the normal levels of Substance P, a neurotransmitter that relays chemical messages about pain in the spinal fluid. There is a large degree of smooth muscle contraction and low serotonin levels (a result of poor sleep). Human growth levels are low, cortisol levels (hormone secreted by the adrenal glands) are high. This eventually depletes the adrenal system. There is also evidence of abnormal brain waves at Stage 4, which is associated with the deepest level of sleep. Poor sleep, in itself, will cause disease in time.

Again, we are confronted with a disease that offers little hope for those with it since a specific cause is unknown. I said that I suspected Mary's trigger was an emotional trauma. The yin or soft element of women is considered more susceptible to emotional damage than the, at least outward, yang element of men, who handle stress totally differently. I learned that Mary's husband left her for his physical therapist after entering rehab to recover from an auto accident. Mary went from being a devoted wife with deep Italian cultural beliefs about home and family, to a woman bedridden and needing a wheelchair. To add insult to injury, after being labeled a chronic pain patient, her insurance benefits were cancelled. Since you probably read the earlier explanation of the toxic chemical brew that gets released during stress or trauma, it is easy to see how the environment for fibromyalgia can be created in individuals. Though protocols to detoxify these by-products and poisons can clear the body, a level of inner work is also needed to clear out toxic emotions. Another example of why I recommend any detoxification program involve body, mind, and spirit.

Patricia

In regard to the many therapies you've read about so far in these case histories, I'd like to add a very special note here. Challenges in life, when embraced with a positive spirit and use of a sincere from-the-heart attempt towards resolution—especially when done with mind, body, heart, and soul—can be enormous opportunities for learning and growth. When a person rises to the occasion and takes on the challenge, magnificent events begin to manifest. The Universe, with all of its power and blessings, steps in. As my dear friend and medicine man from the Shinnecock Indian nation often says, "Faith can move mountains; the rest of us need shovels."

I first got to know Patricia as a patient. She later played a profound role in my life where the experience helped me learn much about love, courage, compassion, faith, and healing. She had an enormous challenge, to say the least. Not that any of us lives like a saint, but her lifestyle and negative connection to an area of work and the persons involved seemed, to me at least, to have poisoned her life in many ways. A casualty, of course, was her health—in every realm.

A doctor "discovered" her cervical cancer at the morbidly progressed third stage level. This is not a good stage to be at and carries a poor prognosis, even with therapy. Facing the prospect of losing everything in life and her death leaving her five-year old son without his mother, she felt devastated and virtually destroyed. When she turned to me for help, I knew I had a formidable challenge, as well. It's not my nature to back away from a challenge, so I embraced it. Practically overnight, I went from being a person with a fair degree of experience in the field of pain management to someone who had to take an unbelievable warp-speed crash course in the Zen of assisting someone back to health and in her case, hopefully life. I kept in mind, The greater the challenge, the greater the reward. Little did I realize this step was the first onto the new path my life would follow.

I went back to the pathology books, back to the basics, and personally prayed quite a bit about this. I consulted other experts and began, at a rapid pace, to enter a crusade to learn everything about cancer care, especially her particular type. Frankly, one cannot learn everything in the field of health, so cancer was a condition that had never been a component of academic allure for me and not my clinical passion. Patricia was adamant about not using conventional medicine and indicated she'd rather die with dignity than waste away, stripped of human form as she'd experienced with those she'd attended to during their last days. This began my milestone journey for which I am eternally grateful.

Tapping into the wisdom of my associates (though I consider them my brothers) at the University of Natural Medicine—Drs. Zhou, Milam, Smith and other colleagues—I proceeded to learn ozone therapy, ultraviolet blood purification therapy (UVB), and deepened my knowledge of Eastern medicine. I began to impart mind-body-spirit healing foundations to her, applied principles of super-nutrition, and got her to Know Sweat. This was, of course, in the form of qigong instruction, heated yoga, meditation, spiritual discussions, sweat that led to detoxing her body—and more sweat. And prayer. It worked. So did the other therapies mentioned here.

Five months of intensive therapies later, and on my daughter's birthday, Patricia experienced a massive purging bleed with the residue of the tumor released from her body. Her GYN indicated a well-healed area of what was formerly an area of massive disease. It was a time of great relief. While Patricia must constantly focus to maintain body-mind-spirit balance, her attitude is a testament to the greatest healer of all time. No, not me by a long shot, but the Almighty or whatever name a person cares to use. And let's not forget the indomitable human spirit, which she demonstrated throughout.

Zen, in practice and *great questioning*, led her (and me) to great answers. This produced great faith which is the mover of mountains, and great courage from which to take action. So to Patricia I say, Thank you for giving me the unconditional faith, courage, and opportunity to tap into the divine knowledge of the infinite so I may carry out the sacred work of healing under His guidance and protection.

These are just several of many, many success stories I could share with you. I've given you insights into various sweat therapies as well as oxygenation, mind-body-spirit, herbal, vitamin, mineral, and enzyme protocols—and probably far more medical terminology than you ever want to digest again. But I want you to have more than just a skim-the-surface understanding of the effects of toxicity on your body and life.

I originally thought I would include in great detail, my ordeal with the medical legal system in this book, but will instead, give you a short summary. It is ongoing, but, I believe, finally beginning to wind down (is it safe to go back into the water?). I decided to share this extraordinary story in an up-coming book entitled, *"Zen and the Legal System."* This book will share my experiences of that system's attempts to crush me in much the same way represented in Steve's story cited earlier and how I used and still use the Zen Warrior Way to cope. However, in the last chapter, I want to offer something of an introduction to this experience so that you learn at least a little of what doctors who use complementary protocols contend with, as well as why it is vital that you deliberately learn all you can to make conscious decisions about how you maintain your health and participate in any healing you may need.

Of course, I follow all the protocols listed in this book, including qigong, meditation, sweat therapy, and sword mastery—written about in my book, *"Zen and the Way of the Sword."* My nature is a high-energy one; but, I keep it at full-throttle by following my own advice. There is so much I want to accomplish in my life, including my goal to contribute to health education on this planet. At this point when people ask me what I do, my first priority is "educator" or conduit for information. Therefore, it is imperative I maintain my health and a level of natural energy that facilitates getting done all that I get done and intend to do.

I do want to share that before my medical legal ordeal began, I was fortunate to meet a Shaolin priest, a Grand Master—Master Tak Wah Eng. We traveled together to the Shaolin Temple in China. Because of him, I am now a Master in Martial Arts. It is because of his guidance, wisdom, prayers, and training that I stayed sane through this ordeal. He taught me to wear the warrior spirit, to be the warrior. To recognize what is important, to practice forgiveness and compassion. He impressed upon me the importance of not harboring hatred, bitterness, or revenge. This amazing man can tap into my emotions—and always be right—based on the odor of my sweat during his grueling Shaolin workouts, and do so from across the room.

His sessions leave me in intense, drenching sweat. Anger and frustration melt away, along with toxic emotions and the poisons they produce in my body. The point of telling you this is that even if we master techniques, even if we detoxify our bodies, we are human beings. We feel pain and hurt. As such, life is an ongoing experience, one we address in every moment. You must never seduce yourself into believing that once you do certain things, you are rid of stress and toxicity forever. That is delusion and unwise. You are a part of a process. You and the process are one.

For all my knowledge and wisdom gained from my many and varied experiences, I credit Master Tak for literally saving my life. Were it not for his guidance through what I consider the most stressful time of my life—yes, even more so than my time in the various war-torn countries I mentioned—the toxicity of my ordeal might have defeated me. I constantly thank God for the helping angels and sages who consistently come into my life, as I am sure come into yours, as well.

I confess to being something of an idealist. My ideal vision is that one day, the medical industry and all health care providers, as well as pharmaceutical and insurance companies will awaken to a higher conscious level, a level where care for fellow members of our human family is sacrosanct and placed above profits. For anyone, in any profession or path in life, I offer this: "Do good, reap good rewards."

"Out there in the spotlight, you're a million miles away;
 and every ounce of energy, you try to give away—
 as the sweat pours out of your body like the music that you play."
Jon English

THE LEGAL MEDICAL SWEAT
THE EXTRAORDINARY EPILOGUE

My spiritual and martial arts brother, Sensei Enzo Aliotta, urged me to add this chapter in my book. Since my legal medical experience caused me to "sweat," it made sense to let you know something about it. However, he suggested I name the chapter, "Personal Indomitable Spirit." I felt his suggestion honored what I had to pull from deep within myself and use in the physical world to survive in a period called "Medical McCarthyism" by some members of the healing arts, and I thank him for that recognition. However, I want the title to easily reflect to readers what this chapter will be about. In a way, I guess it is like Part 2 of the story I conveyed to you earlier. In *"Zen and the Legal System,"* I hope to give you the *final* sequel which will be enveloped by the prayers and blessings of those who are a testament to following at least some of the guidelines I've provided.

As a concert recitalist and orchestral violinist—my original music training, I give my all to the music. I become one with the instrument and the notes. It is the same for me as a healer who has an extensive allopathic and complementary background of certifications and practical experiences. With complete humility, I say that I know myself and my purpose in life to be a healer. In fact, I've managed to therapeutically merge the two. Many doctors I know have a deeply artistic side. Unfortunately, the nature of the work often forces it to be repressed or subjugated. The left brain hemisphere is usually forced to dominate the right in order to perform as a competent medical doctor with all this type of work entails and demands.

Just as a soloist sits in the spotlight so that all attention is focused on him or her, the legal medical system has similarly placed me and others into their own spotlight or, rather, as their target to take aim at. I want to share some of my experience with you now, so that you understand what I and other health care practitioners contend with simultaneous to our dedication to heal and expand our knowledge about restoring health to the whole being.

First, many of you will relate to the fact that most, I'm not claiming all, involved in the allopathic health care system deal with people as statistics, not as individuals. I mentioned earlier that they are given guidelines they are expected to follow or otherwise be penalized. These guidelines come from those who are involved in the monetary aspect of health care. As the statement advises: Follow the money trail.

The *problem* with complementary medicine is

• It addresses each person as an individual who is
  mind-body-emotion-spirit;

• It uses ingredients and elements that are readily found in nature,
  so cannot be patented (for large pharmaceutical profits); and

• Through guidance of a trained health care practitioner, this is
  a more gentle way to heal.

All of these have a common thread: They are cost-effective. If you are a part of the money trail, you want to do whatever generates as much income as you possibly can in order to keep it coming and prevent as much of what you have from going out. A perfect example is back in the 1980s, HMOs decided that when a woman had a mastectomy, this radical surgery should be treated as an out-patient event. They decided it was fine to send a woman home the day of, or if she was lucky, the day after her surgery with the drainage tube still inserted and a bag attached to collect the fluids, with no one qualified to monitor what happened afterwards. Lawsuits from many tragic cases, finally challenged some of these types of atrocities. The negative jokes about HMOs became as prevalent as those about lawyers, i.e., They had more suits than Brooks Brothers.

Complementary medicine has always been around in some form; in fact, it is the original "standard" health care practice. But perhaps the tendencies such as the example above, and other experiences either you or someone you know have had with the allopathic system, propelled certain individuals to look at health care differently. Some decided that perhaps preventative maintenance was a better idea than having to ever deal with the treatment offered by the system. That, perhaps, complementary protocols were either better or, at least, offered an equal chance to heal from disease without the side-effects of allopathic medicines and invasive procedures. And, these individuals were right.

Although the allopathic system was not happy about this, insurance and drug companies—the strange bedfellows of the allopathic system (why leave out their brokers?)—realized the money trail was taking a detour from their pockets into the coffers of complementary health care practitioners, massage therapists, whole-foods nutritionists, and health food stores with shelves of vitamins and other natural remedies. A great deal of pain and suffering was inflicted on chiropractors who after a long fight, which still continues, managed to get the mainstream community to accept the legitimacy of their services. Over the last 25 years, many insurance companies have attempted to modify, though very slightly, their adamant adversity to complementary protocols. Some now pay for massage, chiropractic care, yoga or other more relaxing exercise forms; yet, they still keep tight reins on this. This is where my story picks up.

Somewhere between my colorful days in Turkey, various training programs, and the period of time called "life" where a person makes plans and raises children, I gained extensive training in pain management. I recognized and believed I had the need to make a part of my operations mobile so I could provide services to communities many won't even contemplate driving through at a high rate of speed, much less park and wait. I set up my mobile health care delivery system (complete with diagnostic equipment) with such a commitment to serve, I put my life resources into it. My staff and I went to the poorest neighborhoods and acted as affiliates through medical centers, churches, civic organizations—any group that could lead us to where the people who needed our services were. One side-effect of this for me was I began to develop a fondness for gospel music from the many healing masses I attended and spoke at.

We donated vitamins, food, offered acupuncture, nutritional guidance, pain management, and basic medical services at every opportunity. I successfully merged complementary medicine with mainstream medicine in my area of specialty. If a person had any form of insurance, we accepted it. But many, as might be expected, had no insurance and limited or no income. No one was turned away. I was beginning to feel like I was on top of the world, fulfilling a true purpose.

Apparent by what happened after I began to do this, I must have really peeved off the insurance industry as a result of the expanded degree of care and ultimately what is coined as "over-utilization" in the industry. Roughly translated, this means fees for legitimate patient care, payment for which decreases the bottom line and, ultimately, year-end bonuses for the higher-ups. As I indicated before, any medical service which cuts into the pie is somehow deemed to be "unnecessary," or worse.

One very aggressive insurance investigative company started to probe into my business, my life, and my family. This involved continuous harassment and surveillance. They let this be known publicly so any person even thinking of doing business with me would be frightened away. Not surprisingly, it worked since it did have an major negative impact on my business. This was, in hindsight, also a great experience since it taught me a great deal about "human nature." You learn who your friends are by who remains steadfast at your side. Please see my tribute to the late Dr. Sylvester Leaks in Acknowledgments. Along with Dr. Leaks and Dr. Franklyn Richardson, members of what is called a "minority" community, stood with me, as well. I suppose those persecuted for beliefs or for simply being who they are creates kindred spirits, for which I am eternally grateful. I thank the Universe, everyday, for my cherished friends.

I like to consider myself a compassionate, caring person so one time, went to the two people sitting in a car as they watched my office to see if they would like me to have coffee brought out to them. Even though it was a really cold day, they refused my offer. I walked away wondering if their faces were red from the cold or... Well, that would be speculation.

I first realized there was a problem when the insurance claims for my rendered medical services were refused payment. This caused me to pursue my claims in civil court. The insurance company representatives, listed as experts, were paid to be there to make an argument against any and all treatment. I won the majority; but a great number were lost "in absentia," a reward for some since I was not able to defend them personally, usually as a result of being in remote areas doing some humanitarian work with my University or other good-will organizations. They pitted their IME (independent medical "expert") doctors against me. The vast majority of these are paid character assassins who render an opinion favorable to the party hiring them. Why would they hire them, otherwise? Many do not have practices where they actually treat and heal patients, but get paid to render their *expertise* which is always a well-motivated opinion, generating pages and pages of findings after seeing the patient for no more than three to five minutes. I have had patients actually time these exams!

This did not make the companies happy and I found myself dealing next with one of the most well-organized private insurance investigative companies in the country. My experience with them indicated that they would stop at nothing to avoid payments by the 260+ insurance companies they work for. Their flyers and seminars even boast the claim of their ability to avoid and stop payments to health care practitioners. Can you believe the brazenness? Every doctor is, thus, a crook—according to their twisted logic. This is a little bit different from the pleasant man or woman smiling on the TV ads.

A common tactic used by these private entities that have vast resources, when they believe they cannot win or do not wish to sink their own resources into a process, is to broaden the conflict by bringing the "system" into the fight. What I mean is that they bring the fight to regulatory and enforcement agencies, specifically set up to protect the public from tyranny and terror, to lessen their own financial burden. These agencies, by the way (let's not forget the basics here), were established in accordance with a wonderful, sacred law built on the principles of God, along with a sacred privilege to protect American citizens from tyranny and ensure their ability to pursue life, liberty, and happiness. It's call the *Constitution*. Since many of these agencies have elected representatives (vs. appointed ones), where do you think the funding for their careers come from? Certainly not from children who sell lemonade at health fairs. As you can imagine, this represents a clear conflict of interest. Most doctors, especially those who render care to the most "undeserving" Black, Hispanic, and immigrant communities, get tangled into this nightmare web and become paralyzed in their practices and, ultimately, in their personal lives. Most simply don't have the money, or conviction, to fight these agencies or the system. When you are in the right, I say, "Fight," and with conviction. Use your Zen Warrior Spirit. If you want to believe "you're in good hands," or "we make you part of our family," continue to do so. At your own risk. Survivors of Katrina are still scratching their heads and wondering what went wrong.

Soon, I learned that many of my patients were being subjected to intense questioning by investigators and other officials in what they called "examination under oath." This process actually had a greater semblance to an interrogation in many cases. The sight of an official-looking person with a menacing demeanor, a gun, and badge approaching a poor, unsophisticated person is, to say the least, unnerving. Since most of these patients served by my operation, as well as my mobile unit, were legal and probably illegal aliens and people of color, they knew their situations were jeopardized (as I said, slavery never ends; it just takes on more creative forms). Most were uneducated, not savvy about the system and their rights, and faced the threat of deportation. In fact, incarceration and other unpleasant outcomes were also suggested as remedies for those who did not give the answers required of them. They were terrorized into saying things that were simply, and later proven to be, untrue. I learned it was insinuated that they should state they never received the treatment reported for claim. Even some of my neighbors received anonymous calls in order to get them to provide information about me and were told, "We'll make it worth your while." Fear, when used well, is an awesome weapon. It can coerce, cripple, and destroy. Politicians have used it like a sharp sword throughout history. **To keep one's spirit strong, the mind must be sharper than the opposition's sword.** This method was part of my inspiration to write, *"Zen and the Way of the Sword."*

Rather than focus solely on my healing practice, I now had to get my own team of attorneys and investigators together, as well. My team became this investigative insurance company's worst nightmare. They visited many of the already terrified patients who had been coerced into "confessions" in order to get and document the true story. Because of their efforts, this insurance agency and its investigators were exposed. A settlement was made in my favor, whereby, they asked me to sign a "hold harmless." Never did, never will. The world should know. Actually, their unraveling came when several patients indicated under oath, they had been harrassed so badly that it caused exacerbation of their medical conditions. This is immoral—not to mention a few other things. The very people who were supposed to protect society from medical fraud were the ones perpetrating it. They had to pay me much of what I claimed. As time went on, several senior claims adjustors were "replaced." I think they felt very cheated since they probably expected a huge Christmas bonus and promotion for exposing a "dangerous" person like myself.

But the fun didn't stop here. I got a letter from the State Education Department questioning my professionalism regarding the care of the very same patients cleared. Granted, the purpose of the SED is to make certain licensed professionals practice a "standard of care" that does not harm patients. That's fair and should be done across the board. They also have a department set up to protect the public from harmful practices. That, in itself, is a "whole other issue." The SED alleged that these same patients who were treated and benefitted from the treatment—and as I said, it was later proven they actually received treatment allegedly not received—were complaining about the care they'd received. I don't think so! My team went back into the trenches and discovered none of these patients had *ever* filed a complaint. So where were the complaints coming from? When I demanded to know this before proceeding (which would, of course, explain many confusing mysteries surrounding such cases), the mastodon, once again, retreated into the cave. It sticks its head out intermittently.

Certainly, there should be a safeguard against doctors and practitioners who mistreat or engage in negligent practices with patients and against those who rip off the system. However, my particular situation was instigated by insurance companies that simply did not want to pay what was owed, *not* by unsatisfied or injured patients as was being claimed. This should not be used as a weapon by the insurance industry when they know they have too much of a fight on their hands. I see this pattern repeating consistently with other doctors. At the end of the ordeal, the one truly hurt is (once again) the person who needs the care and, ironically, has paid so he or she can get it.

This process continues in my life on occasion, which causes a good deal of my time to be spent meeting with attorneys and answering questions in court. This kind of practice is one of many that doctors, such as myself, contend with on a regular basis. Some have had their doors closed and their records confiscated. I know several who succumbed to the pressure and took their own lives. The fact that my mind-body-spirit harmony is still strong and I am still here to give you this book is a testament to health-enhancing wisdom—the same wisdom I share here with you. It is a tribute to having practiced what I impart to you—a clear example of "practice what you preach." Under normal circumstances, the stress of this ordeal would easily destroy any person whose three components mentioned, are not in harmony.

Many health care providers simply stopped practicing in these, and other environments, subjecting the already suffering populations to the only "care" they can receive. This usually involves, on average and documented by national statistics, a wait of over 15 hours in an emergency room and usually includes palliative care in the form of pain killers. By the way, the average wait in affluent or middle-class neighborhoods is less than 5 hours.

The people who ostensibly run these companies, routinely show up at social functions with their ultra high-end sports cars and entertain "business associates" on their yachts—tributes to their ill-gotten gains that are flaunted in well-publicized manners like grown-up children. All this lavishness is made possible by the misery and shattered hopes and health they inflict upon their fellow man, and helps to destroy the promise of the "promised land." Without health and trained health care professionals available to protect and foster it, the promise of life, liberty, and the pursuit of happiness—as the great words attest as our right—becomes another pipe-dream, a hollow promise, indeed. I have seen the fallout on the needy sector.

An outsider researching these people would be astounded at all the generous contributions they make to "needy causes." Sure. Why not? Since this excess is cleverly extracted from the same community they feast upon. To the naive, they appear to be true humanitarians. Instead, they are creating the greatest sin against humanity and God— by victimizing those who are already in a great state of suffering.

The use of local, state, and federal government regulatory agencies to further financial ends of a private sector such as the insurance industry (or any other one for that matter), is not only unethical, it crosses over into an extremely questionable realm of legal redress. The issue is, Who has deep enough pockets to pursue it, even if they are right?

An article in the *New York Times* (October 14, 2006) entitled, "Earnings for Insurers are Soaring," is one I recommend you look up. Do you think the smiling and reassuring actor with the hypnotic voice who pitches for the company is the one you'll have to contend with when you or someone you love needs to be compensated? Animals with sharp teeth come into the gladiator's arena when you have to deal with them. This scenario repeats itself over and over, threatening decent doctors, and of course, by attrition, their pursuit of health and happiness.

I am consistently asked to turn over my files for no apparent reason and, thereby, breach my doctor-patient oath of confidentiality—something I continue to refuse to do. And in my case, because of my vows as an ordained minister, since all of these patients also receive spiritual counseling for their trauma and many associated losses, as well, and develop problems they don't wish to see on the front page of a tabloid, it's imperative I maintain my sworn-to confidentiality. It's also a right protected by our Constitution. Every yin has its yang. In a way, I should thank them since they have helped me develop my Zen nature for dealing with problems. In Eastern philosophy, it is said that, "Without enemies, we can never develop strength." So true.

When I took my Hippocratic oath, one of the things I promised was to "first do no harm." To me, this not only means in the treatment and care of every person who entrusts their health to me, but also never to harm them by turning over the sensitive, personal aspects of their records to those who seek to defraud their own system—and mine—

and yours. Contrary to all the suffering and pain (karmic or not), I hold no bitterness or venom about this. Since anger is a double-edged sword, it damages both sides. It is, instead, an education, one that has elevated me to a higher level of spirituality, and perhaps in the end, will allow my story to help others become better people—people who operate more from compassion and consciousness than more typical motivations.

My ideal would be to bring health and well-beingness to every person on the planet. It is an ideal—a feasible ideal I intend to continue to strive towards until it becomes a reality. It is everyone's right as proclaimed in our most sacred document—the Constitution. This assault on my life and profession does not stop me from committing myself and my services to help and educate as many as I can. Another ideal would be to heal the allopathic health care system, the insurance and drug companies, and those affiliated with both groups. That's a far larger challenge. So, I think I'll focus primarily on those individuals who seek what I offer. Whichever side of the equation individuals fall on—patients or those involved in the system—all are members of my human-spiritual family, even those who deem me their "enemy." Because of each of them, my conscious awareness and understanding and compassion continue to grow.

Often, the wealthy and unseen people running such agencies, must undergo a very negative challenging experience that results in another negative experience called pain in order to undergo a paradigm shift. As the laws of karma go, they will have such an experience if they do not amend their ways.

We see such an example in John Newton, the composer of one of the most cherished sacred hymns written, *"Amazing Grace."* As a sea captain who participated in transporting slaves from Sierra Leone, Africa, he was affected after reading Thomas a Kempis', *"Imitation of Christ."* A spiritual and moral awakening began to penetrate his reality when he faced almost certain loss of his ship, cargo, and his own life in a violent storm. When his prayers to be spared were answered, he came to terms with the inhumanity of not only kidnapping human beings, but treating them as cattle (or worse) by laying them side-by-side to maximize space, and chaining them together in the cargo hold (to prevent suicide). It's believed that the general mortality rate of the "cargo" was 20-percent, more if disease broke out. The dead were thrown into the sea. Newton's awareness of such hideous treatment of men, women, and children—different from him in only surface ways, and created by the same God, caused him to abandon such business for profit, become a preacher, and write

Amazing grace, how sweet the sound
That saved a wretch like me,
I once was lost, but now am found,
Was blind, but now I see.

'Twas grace that taught my heart to fear,
And grace my fears relieved.
How precious did that grace appear
The hour I first believed.

Through many dangers, toils and snares,
I have already come.
'Tis grace hath brought me safe thus far,
And grace will lead me home.

One can create "legal laws" that help foster their own cause. They may even break laws, but they can never escape *karmic laws* that guide the universe. The pain and suffering I and others have experienced at the hands of those who aim to destroy us, is something I would never wish on another. Yet, healers such as myself, are not the only ones targeted. Some of the poorest segments of society are seen as feeding grounds by ruthless insurers. By law, you cannot drive a car without insurance—insurance designed to take care of medical needs if you are injured. Yet, if someone needs such care, it becomes a form of hell to attempt to get such care paid for.

Agencies that become "bosom buddies" with insurers, function in a manner that protects their interests. They begin to call the shots, so-to-speak. Follow the money trail. I ask any entity to come forward and prove this is not so. When they demand "discovery" from doctors who've allegedly "erred," equal discovery must be mandated from insurers. But this would reveal their hierarchy, web, or tangled and often obscured relationships, policy influence, and money trail. Such a journey has the potential to reveal illicit, unethical tactics that have questionable legal grounds. This process entering my life has been especially challenging since I am a man whose relatives perished under earlier Russian and Nazi tyranny. I came to the "land of the free," only to have a yoke of terror begin all over again. And all because I seek to heal and ease suffering.

We are forever becoming enlightened and have the responsibility to pass it on. To quote Oliver Wendell Holmes, Sr., again, "Man's mind, once stretched by a new idea, never regains its original dimensions." Because of each of them, as well as every other person who touches my life, I am who I am today. As a Zen practitioner, how can I do anything other than appreciate the gifts they've brought and bring to my life...that is, once my ego-self has a chance to vent and I remember who I know myself to be. Even a Master must not repress true emotions and make his body-mind-spirit toxic. I do not claim to be a Master, but I do claim to be on a path of mastery—of my self—on all levels.

As Mr. Spock would say, "Live long, and prosper."
And, do so in good health.

Om mani padme hum.

ABOUT THE AUTHOR

Bill Akpinar may have a string of letters after his name and a list of ongoing accomplishments that make a person wonder if this man has more than 24 hours in a day, but that's not the most impressive thing about him. What is impressive is that he is like a force of nature. Combine a force of nature with a purpose and the result is quite dynamic. Dr. Bill's purpose: To do anything within his power to help his fellow man restore and maintain well-being of body, mind, and spirit.

Bill doesn't offer any guidance on these three levels that is theoretical. It's all based on personal experience. As you keep reading this abbreviated biography, you'll see credentials and other information that demonstrate a passion for arts, sciences, and humanity. Hopefully, you'll also see the warrior who does not live solely or mostly in his mind, but treats life as a banquet. Bill doesn't simply ingest and assimilate information and moments in life, but absorbs and becomes one with them.

Medical:
• Four Doctorate degrees: M.D. (Physician), D.D.S. (Dentist), Dr.Ac. (Acupuncture), Ph.D. (Pain Management and Oriental Medicine)

• Numerous Board Certifications and Fellowships including Pain Management, Anesthesiology, Forensic Dentistry, Acupuncture, Traumatic Stress—to name just a few
• Certified Forensic Medical Investigator

Other Positions Held:
• Medical Director at the Center for Healing, Queens, NY — Practices and teaches healing arts to students and doctors who rotate through his clinic
• Institutional Board of Chancellors and Director of the World Organization of Natural Medicine
• Dean and Medical Director of the University of Natural Medicine (focusing on global health problems and education)
• Served as Assistant Professor of Pain Management and Anesthesiology — New York College of Podiatry, New York City
• Established pain-mitigation programs at the Lutheran Medical Center in New York City, L.I.J./Hillside Medical Center, and Bronx Lebanon Hospital
• Served as Medical and Nutritional Constultant to St. John's University's "Red Storm" basketball team
• Physician for the U.S. International Karate team under Master Tokey Hill

Travel and Lectures:
• Lectures in areas of expertise, including his approach to integrative medicine, to health care practitioners around the world.
•Keynote Speaker to 2,000-plus doctors for Moscow's Russian Society for Natural Medicine (Feb. 2002) — subsequently awarded Honorary Doctor of Natural Medicine by this Society
• Lectures and teaches healing arts at U.S. and international facilities
• Keynote Speaker, First International Ozone Conference — Istanbul, Turkey (2006)

Programs and Projects:
• Eric Clapton's "Crossroads Progam" in Antigua — a unique, advanced state-of-technology to treat children and adults with addictive personalities and addictive disorders — established the protocols and trained staff in Qigong and acupuncture to heal addictions
• Founder of *Doctors with a Vision* — Global mission of World Peace Through World Health — "This vision requires a sufficient number of others to reach critical mass necessary to bring about physical, mental, and spiritual health."

Additional Training:
• Advanced specialized healing arts with the personal physician of the Dalai Lama in Tibet
• Many years of personal martial arts training with former U.S. and World Karate Champion Terrence "Tokey" Hill; world-renowned Judo and Jujitsu Master, Jack Krystek; and Grandmaster Tak Wah Eng—author, martial arts master, and swordmaster—who helped shape the form and style of Chinese martial arts including the use of weapons
• Martial body and mind training in People's Republic of China (mainland), Republic of China (Taiwan), Tibet, and other venues
• Ordained Taoist and Buddhist Minister

Other:
• Teaches martial and healing arts including Taijiquan, Qigong, and Shotokan Karate
• Frequent guest speaker on radio and television talk shows in the U.S. and China.
• Multi-instrumental musician
• Former concert recitalist and orchestral violinist
• Prolific author
• Many more accomplishments than will be listed here
• His greatest lifetime accomplishment — father of Adam and Melissa

Add the fact of Bill's genuine caring for his fellow man to his vast wealth of experience and knowledge, and you may understand why it is my greatest pleasure and privilege to work with him. Each project we work on evidences him as a man with a mission and the means to make a difference. Bill Akpinar is a true spiritual warrior who dedicates his life in service to others.

Joyce Shafer
Editor

ACKNOWLEDGMENTS

My grandfather, Abdulhamit Yorga, who was instrumental in developing my curiosity for learning and reading—often by "bribing" me to the tune of a dollar for every book I read—which worked! He was a tough soul, yet a true inspiration. The pain inflicted upon him by the Russians and Nazis in World War II never dulled his sense of compassion. He is one man whose spirit should continue to live after the third generation. My grandmother, Emine Yorga, an example of human caring, compassion, and love for any soul whom she happened to encounter. She would feed the many stragglers and strangers I brought home without bothering to ask me who they were.

My parents, for helping me develop into the man I am today, despite their own personal hardships, not to mention the countless hardships I, myself, imposed on them during the period of my youth! My family, for giving me support through all my different searches—paths which may have appeared neurotic to a non-searcher.

My teachers, who in their own frame of reference—even if perhaps limited—and in the only way they knew, tried to instill the sense of right and wrong despite their own inner conflicts they were forced to deal with at the time. I assure you they gave the best they had.

My patients and persons who placed the supreme, unconditional faith in my ability to help them as a doctor, minister, and healer. Despite the fact that doctor literally means *teacher*, they continue to remain *my* teachers. I thank you for your faith and the opportunities you have given me. For those whose outcomes may not have been as anticipated, I beg forgiveness and offer prayer. Only God is the true healer. Everything I gave was given with heart, mind, and spirit all of the time.

My martial arts teachers and dear friends, Terrence "Tokey" Hill, Jack Krystek, Giuseppe and Enzo Aliotta. You helped instill the spirit of the Zen warrior in myself and my children. The special individuals who taught me about compassion, love, and caring. You know who you are! Joyce Shafer, for her invaluable help and inspiration in helping to bring the thoughts and ideas together in such a wonderful way. Spencer Bagley, for his endless creative genius and talent in continuing to bring it all together. Janet Hanchey, for her remarkable renderings that brought another dimension to the book.

Persons and entities whose faces I may never know in the insurance, regulatory, licensing, and other organizations, for your crusade to discredit and destroy my name, career, family, and spirit. No one who is mainstream likes trail blazers. You also know who you are. I hope this book serves as a starting point for reassessment of your ways and, hopefully, the beginning of your own enlightenment. Yes, thank you. You have forged the way for me to develop the Zen warrior spirit and furthered my resolve to help and champion for the underdog! I now understand, much more clearly, the plight of those who have nowhere to turn in times of trouble. It taught me that human enslavement never quite ends. It just takes on more creative forms as we "evolve."

My late cherished friend—"Dad"—a mighty warrior with mighty intellect, Dr. Sylvester Leaks, who was there for me in all of the pain, tur-

Contact Dr. Bill Akpinar at drakpinar@aol.com.
(Please note "No Sweat" in the Subject line.)

SUGGESTED READING

A Cure for All Diseases. Dr. Hulda Regehr Clark

Alternative Medicine: The Definitive Guide.
Burton Goldberg, John W. Anderson, and Larry Trivieri

A Practical Guide to Vibrational Medicine:
Energy Healing and Spiritual Transformation
Richard Gerber, M.D.

Detoxify or Die. Sherry A. Rogers

Disease Prevention and Treatment. Life Extension Foundation

Harrison's Principles of Internal Medicine
Dennis L. Kasper, Eugene Braunwald, Anthony Fauci, and Stephen Hauser

How to Get Well. Ph.D., N.D., Paavo Ariola and M.D. H. Rudolph Alsleben

The Life Extension Revolution:
The New Science of Growing Older Without Aging
Philip Lee Miller and Monica Reinagel

The Merck Manual of Diagnosis and Therapy
Mark H. Beers, Robert S. Porter, and Thomas V. Jones

The Miracle of Fasting: Proven Throughout History for Physical, Mental,
and Spiritual Rejuvenation. Paul C. Bragg and Patricia Bragg

Myofascial Pain and Dysfunction: The Trigger Point Manual
Janet G. Travell, M.D. and David G. Simons, M.D.

Natural Cures "They" Don't Want You to Know About. Kevin Trudeau

Ozone: the eternal purifier of the earth and cleanser of all living beings: the future of ozone in medicine, environment, and society or 21st century medicine and technology now. H. E. Satori

Pathologic Basis of Disease
Stanley L. Robbins, Ramzi S. Cotran, and Vinay Kumar

Pathophysiology. Lee-Ellen Copstead and Jacquelyn Banasik

Prescription for Nutritional Healing. Phyllis A. Balch and James F. Balch

Prostate Health in 90 Days (without drugs or surgery)
Larry Clapp, Ph.D., J.D.

The Secret Life of Water. Masaru Emoto

Shaolin Yoga: Qigong. Dr. Bill Akpinar

Spiritual Nutrition and the Rainbow Diet. Gabriel Cousens, M.D.

Sweat: The Illustrated History and Description of the Finnish Sauna, Russian Bania, Islamic Hamman, Japanese Mushi-Buro, Mexican Temescal, and American Indian and Eskimo Sweatlodge. Mikkel Aaland

Textbook of Medical Physiology. Arthur C. Guyton and John E. Hall

Worldwide Secrets for Staying Young. Paavo Airola

Zen and the Way of the Sword. Dr. Bill Akpinar

APPENDIX

The following information is according to the International Hyperhidrosis Society; its entirety copied as provided on their website (www.SweatHelp.org).

Diseases and Conditions that Can Cause Diaphoresis

A large number of diseases and medical conditions can cause diaphoresis (excess perspiration or sweating). Some of the following diseases and medical conditions are common and their names may be easily recognized even by the non-physician. Others are more rare or obscure. This list is provided as a resource and a service. It is not exhaustive and is in no way meant to replace consultation with a medical professional. Although sweating is a known side effect of the conditions listed below, only a percentage of people affected by these conditions may experience undue sweating. This percentage may vary greatly.

Common Diseases/Conditions
Acute Febrile Illness (e.g., infection)
Alcoholism
Diabetes Mellitus
Gout
Heart Failure
Hyperthyroidism
Lymphoma
Menopause
Obesity
Parkinson's disease
Pregnancy
Rheumatoid arthritis

Nervous System Mediated Conditions
Cortical Condition (mediated by the cerebral cortex)
Congenital autonomic dysfunction with universal pain loss
Congenital ichthyosiform erythroderma
Epidermolysis bullosa simplex
Familial dysautonomia
Gopalan's syndrome
Palmoplantar keratodermas
Pachyonychia congenita (Jadassohn-Lewandowsky syndrome)
Pressure and postural hyperhidrosis
Nail-patella syndrome

Hypothalamic Conditions (mediated by the hypothalamus)
Acute infection
Alcoholism
Carcinoid syndrome
Cardiac shock
Chediak-Higashi syndrome
Chronic arsenic intoxication
Chronic infection (e.g., tuberculosis, malaria, brucellosis)
Cold injury
Debility
Diabetes mellitus
Drug addiction (e.g., cocaine, amphetamines)
Drugs
Familial dysautonomia
Erythrocyanosis
Essential hyperhidrosis
Exercise
Gout
Heart failure (congestive heart failure)
Hines-Bannick syndrome

Hyperpituitarism
Hyperthyroidism
Hypoglycemia
Hypothalamic mass (e.g., tumor, abscess)
Idiopathic unilateral circumscribed hyperhidrosis
Infantile scurvy
Lymphoma
Menopause
Obesity
Parkinson's disease
Pheochromocytoma
Phenylketonuria
POEMS syndrome
Porphyria
Post-enchephalitis
Pregnancy
Pressure and postural hyperhidrosis
Raynaud's phenomenon or disease
Reflex sympathetic dystrophy
Rheumatoid arthritis
Rickets
Stroke/cerebrovascular accident/transient ischemic attack (affecting hypothalamus)
Symmetric lividity of the palms and soles
Vitiligo

Medullary/Spinal Conditions
(mediated by the medulla oblongata or spinal nerves)
Auriculotemporal syndrome
Encephalitis
Granulosis rubra nasi
Physiologic gustatory sweating

Post-traumatic
(spinal cord transaction or thoracic sympathetic chain injury)
Syringomyelia
Tabes dorsalis

Peripheral-Reflexive Conditions
Drugs/medications
Perilsional (e.g., burn)

Non-Neural Conditions
Arteriovenous fistula
Blue rubber bleb nevus syndrome
Cold erythema
Drugs
Glomus tumors
Klippel-Trenaunay syndrome
Local heat
Maffucci's syndrome
Organoid and sudoriparous nevi

THIS LIST IS ADAPTED FROM: HURLEY, H. J., DISEASES OF THE ECCRINE SWEAT GLANDS. IN: BOLOGNIA, J. L., JORIZZO, J.L., RAPHINI, R. P., ET AL (EDS.) DERMATOLOGY, SPAIN: MOSBY, 2001; CHAPTER 41

Drugs/Medications Known to Cause Diaphoresis

Certain prescription and non-prescription medications can cause diaphoresis (excess perspiration or sweating) as a side effect. A list of potentially sweat-inducing medications is provided below. (My note: Now you know what can be done about removing their unnecessary metabolites from the body after their work has been completed.) Medications are listed alphabetically by generic name. U.S. brand names are given in parentheses, if applicable. This list is provided as a resource and a service. It is not exhaustive and is in no way meant to replace consultation with a medical professional. Although sweating is a known side effect of the medications listed below, in most cases only a small percentage of people using the medicines experience undue sweating (in some cases less than 1%). Medications noted with an "*" are the most likely to cause sweating and the frequency of sweating as a side effect from these medications may be as high as 50%.

Abciximab (ReoPro®)
Acamprosate (Campral®)
Acetaminophen and Tramadol (Ultracet™)
Acetophenazine (NA)
Acetylcholine (Miochol-E®)
Acetylcysteine (Acetadote®)
Acitretin (Soriatane®)
Acrivastine and Pseudoephedrine (Semprex® -D)
Acyclovir (Zovirax®)
Adenosine (Adenocard® ; Adenoscan®)
Alemtuzumab (Campath®)
Almotriptan (Axert™)
Alosetron (Lotronex®)
Ambenonium (Mytelase®)
Amitriptyline (Elavil®)

Amlodipine (Norvasc®)

Amoxapine (NA)

Amphotericin B (Liposomal) (AmBisome®)

Anastrozole (Arimidex®)

Anidulafungin (Eraxis™)

Antihemophilic Factor (Recombinant) (Advate; Helixate® FS; Kogenate® FS; Recombinate™; ReFacto®)

Antithymocyte Globulin (Equine) (Atgam®)

Antithymocyte Globulin (Rabbit) (Thymoglobulin®)

Apomorphine (Apokyn™)

Aprepitant (Emend®)

Aripiprazole (Abilify®)

Arsenic Trioxide (Trisenox™)

Atazanavir (Reyataz®)

Atomoxetine (Strattera®)

Atovaquone (Mepron®)

Azacitidine (Vidaza™)

Aztreonam (Azactam®)

Bacitracin (AK-Tracin® [DSC]; Baciguent® [OTC]; BaciiM®)

Baclofen (Lioresal®)

Benazepril (Lotensin®)

Betamethasone (Beta-Val®; Celestone® Soluspan®; Celestone®; Diprolene® AF; Diprolene®; Luxiq®; Maxivate®)

Bethanechol (Urecholine®)

Bexarotene (Targretin®)

Bicalutamide (Casodex®)

Bretylium [DSC] (NA)

Bumetanide (Bumex®)

Buprenorphine (Buprenex®; Subutex®)

Buprenorphine and Naloxone (Suboxone®)

BusPIRone (BuSpar®)

Butorphanol (Stadol®)

Calcitonin (Fortical®; Miacalcin®)

Candesartan (Atacand®)

Candesartan and Hydrochlorothiazide (Atacand HCT™)

Capecitabine (Xeloda®)

Carbachol (Carbastat® [DSC]; Isopto® Carbachol; Miostat®)

Carbamazepine (Carbatrol®; Epitol®; Equetro™; Tegretol ®-XR; Tegretol®)

Carvediol (Coreg®)

Caspofungin (Cancidas®)

Cefditoren (Spectracef™)

Ceftriaxone (Rocephin®)

Celecoxib (Celebrex®)

Cevimeline (Evoxac®)

Cidofovir (Vistide®)

Ciprofloxacin (Apo-Ciproflox®; Ciloxan®; Cipro® XL; Cipro®; CO Ciprofloxacin; Gen-Ciprofloxacin; Novo-Ciprofloxacin; PMS-Ciprofloxacin; ratio-Ciprofloxacin; Rhoxal-ciprofloxacin)

Citalopram (Celexa®)

Cladribine (Leustatin®)

ClomiPRAMINE (Anafranil®)

Clozapine (Clozaril®; FazaClo®)

CycloSPORINE (Gengraf®; Neoral®; Restasis™; Sandimmune®)

Cytomegalovirus Immune Globulin (Intravenous-Human) (CytoGam®)

Daclizumab (Zenapax®)

Danazol (Danocrine® [DSC])

*Desipramine (Norpramin®)

Dextroamphetamine and Amphetamine (Adderall XR®; Adderall®)

Diflunisal (Dolobid® [DSC])

Digoxin (Digitek®; Lanoxicaps®; Lanoxin®)

Dihydroergotamine (D.H.E. 45®; Migranal®)

Diphenoxylate and Atropine (Lomotil®; Lonox®)

Dipyridamole (Persantine®)

Dirithromycin (Dynabac® [DSC])

Dofetilide (Tikosyn™)

Dolasetron (Anzemet®)

Donepezil (Aricept® ODT; Aricept®)

Doxapram (Dopram®)

Doxazosin (Cardura®)

Doxepin (Prudoxin™; Sinequan® [DSC]; Zonalon®)

DOXOrubicin (Liposomal) (Doxil®)

Dronabinol (Marinol®)

Duloxetine (Bymbalta®)

Echothiophate Iodide (Phospholine Iodide®)

Edrophonium (Enlon®; Reversol®)

Efavirenz (Sustiva®)

Eletriptan (Relpax®)

Enalapril (Vasotec®)

Entacapone (Comtan®)

Ephedrine (Pretz-D® [OTC])

Epinephrine (Adrenalin®; EpiPen® Jr; EpiPen®; Primatene® Mist [OTC]; Raphon [OTC]; S2® [OTC]; Twinject™)

Epoprostenol (Flolan®)

Eprosartan (Teveten®)

Ergonovine (NA)

Escitalopram (Lexapro®)

Esmolol (Brevibloc®)

Estazolam (ProSom®)

Eszopiclone (Lunesta™)

Etoposide (Toposar®; VePesid®)

Etoposide Phosphate (Etopophos®)

Exemestane (Aromasin®)

Exenatide (Byetta™)

Fat Emulsion (Intralipid®; Liposyn® III)

Fenofibrate (Antara™; Lipofen™; Lofibra™; TriCor®; Triglide™)

Fentanyl (Actiq®; Duragesic®; Sublimaze®)

Ferric Gluconate (Ferrlecit®)

Fludrocortisone (Florinef®)

Fludrocortisone (Florinef®)

Flumazenil (Anexate®; Romazicon®)

Flunisolide (AeroBid®-M; AeroBid®; Nasarel®)

Fluoxetine (Prozac® Weekly™; Prozac®; Sarafem®)

Flupenthioxol (NA)

Flurazepam (Dalmane®)

Fluticasone and Salmeterol (Advair Diskus®)

Fluvoxamine (NA)

Fomivirsen (Vitravene™ [DSC])

Foscarnet (Foscavir®)

Frovatriptan (Frova®)

Fulvestrant (Faslodex®)

Gadopentetate Dimeglumine (Magnevist®)

Gatifloxacin (Tequin ®; Zymar™)

Glatiramer Acetate (Copaxone®)

GlipiZIDE (Glucotrol® XL; Glucotrol®)

Goserelin (Zoladex®)

Guanfacine (Tenex®)

Haloperidol (Haldol® Decanoate; Haldol®)

Hepatitis A Inactivated and Hepatitis B (Recombinant) Vaccine (Twinrix®)

Hepatitis B Vaccine (Engerix-B®; Recombivax HB®)

Histrelin (Vantas™)

HydrALAZINE (NA)

Hydrocodone and Acetaminophen (Anexsia®; Bancap HC®; Ceta-Plus®; Co-Gesic®; Hycet™; Lorcet® 10/650; Lorcet® Plus; Lorcet®-HD [DSC]; Lortab®; Margesic® H; Maxidone™; Norco®; Stagesic®; Vicodin® ES; Vicodin® HP; Vicodin®; Zydone®)

Ibritumomab (Zevalin®)

Imipramine (Tofranil-PM®; Tofranil®)

Immune Globulin (Intravenous) (Carimune™ NF; Gammagard®

Liquid; Gammagard® S/D; Gammar®-P I.V.; Gamunex®; Iveegam EN; Octagam®; Panglobulin® NF; Polygam® S/D)

Indocyanine Green (IC-Green®)

Infliximab (Remicade®)

Insulin Inhalation (Exubera®)

Insulin Regular (Humulin® R (Concentrated) U-500; Humulin® R; Novolin® R)

Interferon Alfa-2a (Roferon-A®)

Interferon Alfa-2b (Intron® A)

Interferon Alfa-n3 (Alferon® N)

Interferon Alfacon-1 (Infergen®)

Interferon Beta-1b (Betaseron®)

Iodixanol (Visipaque™)

Ipratropium and Albuterol (Combivent®; DuoNeb™)

Irinotecan (Camptosar®)

Iron Dextran Complex (Dexferrum®; INFeD®)

Iron Supplements (Parenteral) (Dexferrum®; Ferrlecit®; INFeD®; Venofer®)

Isoproterenol (Isuprel®)

Isosorbide Dinitrate and Hydralazine (BiDil®)

Isotretinoin (Accutane®; Amnesteem™; Claravis™; Sotret®)

Ketorolac (Acular LS™; Acular® PF; Acular®; Toradol®)

Labetalol (Trandate®)

Leflunomide (Arava®)

Lenalidomide (Revlimid®)

Letrozole (Femara®)

Leuprolide (Eligard®; Lupron Depot-Ped®; Lupron Depot®; Lupron®; Viadur®)

Levalbuterol (Xopenex HFA™; Xopenex®)

Levobupivacaine (Chirocaine® [DSC])

Levodopa and Carbidopa (Parcopa™; Sinemet® CR; Sinemet®)

Levothyroxine (Levothroid®; Levoxyl®; Synthroid®; Unithroid®)

Lidocaine and Epinephrine (LidoSite™; Xylocaine® MPF With Epinephrine; Xylocaine® With Epinephrine)

Liothyronine (Cytomel®; Triostat®)

Liotrix (Thyrolar®)

Lisinopril (Prinivil®; Zestril®)

Lopinavir and Ritonavir (Kaletra®)

Loratadine (Apo-Loratadine®; Claritin® Kids; Claritin®)

Losartan (Cozaar®)

Maprotiline (NA)

Mechlorethamine (Mustargen®)

MedroxyPROGESTERone (Depo-Provera® Contraceptive; Depo-Provera®; depo-subQ provera 104™; Provera®)

Mefloquine (Lariam®)

Megestrol (Megace® ES; Megace®)

Melphalan (Alkeran®)

Mepivacaine (Carbocaine®; Polocaine® Dental; Polocaine® MPF; Polocaine®)

Mepivacaine (Dental) (Carbocaine®; Polocaine®)

Mepivacaine and Levonordefrin (Carbocaine® 2% with Neo-Cobefrin®)

Meropenem (Merrem® I.V.)

Mesalamine (Asacol®; Canasa™; Pentasa®; Rowasa®)

Metaproterenol (Alupent®)

Methadone (Dolophine®; Methadone Diskets®; Methadone Intensol™; Methadose®)

Methotrimeprazine (NA)

Methylene Blue (Urolen Blue®)

Methylergonovine (Methergine®)

Metoprolol and Hydrochlorothiazide (Lopressor HCT®)

Mexiletine (Mexitil® [DSC])

Misoprostol (Cytotec®)

Moclobemide (NA)

Modafinil (Alertec®; Provigil®)

Morphine Sulfate (Astramorph/PF™; Avinza®; DepoDur™; Duramorph®; Infumorph®; Kadian®; MS Contin®; Oramorph SR®; RMS®; Roxanol 100™; Roxanol™-T [DSC]; Roxanol™)

Moxifloxacin (Avelox® I.V.;Avelox®; Vigamox™)

Muromonab-CD3 (Orthoclone OKT® 3)

Mycophenolate (CellCept®; Myfortic®)

Nabumetone (Relafen®)

Nalbuphine (Nubain®)

Naloxone (Narcan® [DSC])

Naphazoline and Antazoline (Vasocon®-A [OTC] [DSC])

Naproxen (Aleve® [OTC]; Anaprox® DS; Anaprox®; EC-Naprosyn®; Midol® Extended Relief; Naprelan®; Naprosyn®; Pamprin® Maximum Strength All-Day Relief [OTC])

Nelfinavir (Viracept®)

Neostigmine (Prostigmin®)

Nesiritide (Natrecor®)

Niacin (Nicor®; Niaspan®; Slo-Niacin® [OTC])

NiCARdipine (Cardene® I.V.; Cardene® SR; Cardene®)

Nicotine (Commit™ [OTC]; NicoDerm® CQ® [OTC]; Nicorette® [OTC]; Nicotrol® Inhaler; Nicotrol® NS; Nicotrol® Patch [OTC])

NIFEdipine (Adalat® CC; Afeditab™ CR; Nefediac™ CC; Nifedical™ XL; Procardia XL®; Procardia®)

Nilutamide (Nilandron®)

Nimodipine (Nimotop®)

Nisoldipine (Sular®)

Nitazoxanide (Alinia®)

Nitroprusside (Nitropress®)

Norepinephrine (Levophed®)

*Nortriptyline (Pamelor®)

Octreotide (Sandostatin LAR®; Sandostatin®)

Olanzapine (Zyprexa® Zydis®; Zyprexa®)

Omeprazole (Prilosec OTC™ [OTC]; Prilosec®)

Omeprazole and Sodium Bicarbonate (Zegerid®)

Oxprenolol (NA)

Oxycodone (OxyContin®; Oxydose™; OxyFast®; OxyIR®; Roxicodone™ Intensol™; Roxicodone™)

Oxycodone and Ibuprofen (Combunox™)

Oxymetazoline (4Way® 12 Hour [OTC]; Afrin® Extra Moisturizing [OTC]; Afrin® Original [OTC]; Afrin® Severe Congestion [OTC]; Afrin® Sinus [OTC]; Duramist® Plus [OTC]; Duration® [OTC]; Genasal [OTC];Neo-Synephrine® 12 Hour Extra Moisturizing [OTC]; Neo-Synephrine® 12 Hour [OTC]; NRS® [OTC]; N_strilla® [OTC]; Vicks Sinex® 12 Hour Ultrafine Mist [OTC]; Vicks Sinex® 12-Hour [OTC]; Visine® L.R. [OTC])

Papaverine (Para-Time SR®)

Paroxetine (Paxil CR®; Paxil®; Pexeva®)

Peginterferon Alfa-2a (Pegasys®)

Peginterferon Alfa-2b (PEG-Intron®)

Pentazocine (Talwin® NX; Talwin®)

Pentaxocine and Acetaminophen (Talcacen®)

Perflutren Lipid Microspheres (Definity®)

Pericyazine (Neuleptil®)

Perindopril Erbumine (Aceon®)

Perphenazine (NA)

Phendimetrazine (Bontril PDM®; Bontril® Slow-Release; Melfiat®; Obezine® [DSC]; Prelu-2® [DSC])

Phenelzine (Nardil®)

Physostigmine (NA)

Phytonadione (Mephyton®)

*Pilocarpine (Isopto® Carpine; Pilopine HS®; Salagen®)

Pimozide (Orap®)

Piperacillin and Tazobactam Sodium (Zosyn®)

Pipotiazine (NA)

Pirbuterol (Maxair™ Autohaler™)

Prazepam (NA)

Praziquantel (Biltricide®)

PrednisoLONE (AK-Pred®; Bubbli-Pred™ [DSC]; Econopred® Plus; Orapred®; Pediapred®; Pred Forte®; Pred Mild®; Prelone®)

Prilocaine (Citanest® Plain)

Prilocaine and Epinephrine (Citanest® Forte Dental)

Prochlorperazine (Compro™)

Propafenone (Rythmol® SR; Rythmol®)

Proparacaine (Alcaine®; Ophthetic®)

Protirelin (Thyrel® TRH [DSC])

*Protriptyline (Vivactil®)

Pseudoephedrine (Biofed [OTC]; Contact® Cold [OTC]; Demetapp® 12-Hour Non-Drowsy Extentabs® [OTC]; Dimetapp® Decongestant Infant [OTC]; ElixSure™ Congestion [OTC]; Genaphed® [OTC]; Kidkare Decongestant [OTC]; Kodet SE [OTC]; Oranyl [OTC]; PediaCare® [OTC]; Sudafed® 24 Hour [OTC]; Sudafed® Children's [OTC]; Sudafed® [OTC]; Sudo-Tab® [OTC]; Sudodrin [OTC]; SudoGest [OTC])

Pyridostigmine (Mestinon® Timespan®; Mestinon®; Regonol®)

Quetiapine (Seroquel®)

Quinapril (Accupril®)

Quinapril and Hydrochlorothiazide (Accuretic®; Quinaretic)

Quinupristin and Dalfopristin (Synercid®)

Rabeprazole (AcipHex®)

Raloxifene (Evista®)

Raltitrexed (NA)

Ramipril (Altace®)

Rho(D) Immune Globulin (BayRho-D® Full-Dose; BayRho-D® Mini-Dose; MICRhoGAM® ; RhoGAM®; Rhophylac®; WinRho® SDF)

Ribavirin (Copegus®; Rebetol®; Ribasphere™; Virazole®)

Ritonavir (Norvir®)

Rivastigmine (Exelon®)

Rizatriptan (Maxalt-MLT®; Maxalt®)

Rofecoxib (Vioxx® [DSC])

Ropinirole (Requip®)

Secretin (SecreFlo™)

Selegiline (Eldepryl®; Emsam®)

Selenium (Selenicaps [OTC]; Selenimin [OTC]; Selepen®)

Selenium Sulfide (Exsel® [DSC]; Head & Shoulders® Intensive Treatment [OTC]; Selsun Blue® 2-in-1 Treatment [OTC]; Selsun Blue® Balanced Treatment [OTC]; Selsun Blue® Medicated Treatment [OTC]; Selsun Blue® Moisturizing Treatment [OTC]; Selsun®)

Sertraline (Zoloft®)

Sibutramine (Meridia®)

Sincalide (Ukinevac®)

Sirolimus (Rapamune®)

Sodium Oxybate (Xyrem®)

Somatropin (Genotropin Miniquick®; Genotropin®; Humatrope®; Norditropin® NordiFlex®; Norditropin®; Nutropin AQ®; Nutropin®; Saizen®; Serostim®; Tev-Tropin™; Zorbtive™)

Sotalol (Betapace AF®; Betapace®; Sorine®)

Streptokinase (Streptase®)

Sumatriptan (Imitrex®)

Tacrolimus (Prograf®; Protopic®)

Tadalafil (Cialis®)

Tamoxifen (Nolvadex® [DSC]; Soltamox™)

Tegaserod (Zelnorm®)

Telithromycin (Ketek®)

Telmisartan (Micardis®)

Telmisartan and Hydrochlorothiazide (Micardis® HCT)

Temazepam (Restoril®)

Tenofovir (Viread®)

Terbutaline (Brethine®)

Testosterone (Androderm®; AndroGel®; Delatestryl®; Depo®-

Testosterone; First® Testosterone MC; First® Testosterone; Striant®; Testim®; Testopel®)

Thalidomide (Thalomid®)

Thiothixene (Navane®)

Thyroid (Armour® Thyroid; Nature-Throid® NT; Westhroid®)

Tiagabine (Gabitril®)

Tigecycline (Tygacil™)

Tinidazole (Tindamax™)

Tirofiban (Aggrastat®)

Tocainide (Tonocard® [DSC])

Tolcapone (Tasmar®)

Topiramate (Topamax®)

Toremifene (Fareston®)

Tositumomab and Iodine I 131 Tositumomab (131 I Anti-B1 Antibody; 131 I-Anti-B1 Monoclonal Antibody; Anti-CD20-Murine Monoclonal Antibody I-131; B1 Antibody; B1; Iodine I 131 Tositumomab and Tositumomab; Tositumomab I-131)

*Trace Metals (Iodopen®; M.T.E.-4®; M.T.E.-5®; M.T.E.-6®; M.T.E.-7®; Molypen®; Multitrace™-4 Neonatal; Multitrace ™-4 Pediatric; Multitrace™-4; Multitrace™-5; Neotrace-4®; P.T.E.-4®; P.T.E.-5®; Pedtrace-4®; Selepen®)

Tramadol (Ultram® ER; Ultram®)

Tranylcypromine (Parnate®)

Tretinoin (Oral) (Vesanoid®)

Triamcinolone (Aristocort® A; Aristocort®; Aristospan®; Azmacort®; Kenalog-10®; Kenalog-40®; Kenalog®; Nasacort® AQ; Tri-Nasal®; Triderm®)

Triprolidine and Pseudoephedrine (Actified® Cold and Allergy [OTC]; Allerfrim® [OTC]; Aphedrid™ [OTC]; Aprodine® [OTC]; Genac® [OTC]; Silafed® [OTC]; Sudafed® Sinus Nighttime [OTC]; Tri-Sudo® [OTC]

Triprolidine, Pseudoephedrine, and Codeine (Triacin-C® [DSC])

Urokinase (Abbokinase® [DSC])

Vaccinia Immune Globulin (Intravenous) (CNJ-016™)

Vardenafil (Levitra®)

Vasopressin (Pitressin®)

Venlafaxine (Effexor® XR; Effexor®)

Vasopressin (Pitressin®)

Verapamil (Calan® SR; Calan®; Covera-HS®; Iosptin® SR; Verelan® PM; Verelan®)

Xylometazoline (Otrivin® Pediatric [OTC] [DSC]; Otrivin® [OTC] [DSC])

Yohimbine (Aphrodyne®; Yocon®)

Ziconotide (Prialt®)

Zidovudine (Retrovir®)

*Zinc Supplements (Cold-Eeze® [OTC]; Galzin™; Orazinc® [OTC]; Zincate®)

Ziprasidone (Geodon®)

Zolmitriptan (Zomig-ZMT™; Zomig®)

Zolpidem (Ambien CR™; Ambien®)

Zonisamide (Zonegran®)

Zopiclone (NA)

Zuclopenthixol (NA)

* = known to commonly cause diaphoresis

REFERENCE: LEXI-DRUGS DATABASE, THE OFFICIAL DRUG REFERENCE OF THE AMERICAN PHARMACISTS ASSOCIATION, THE NATIONAL PROFESSIONAL SOCIETY OF PHARMACISTS.

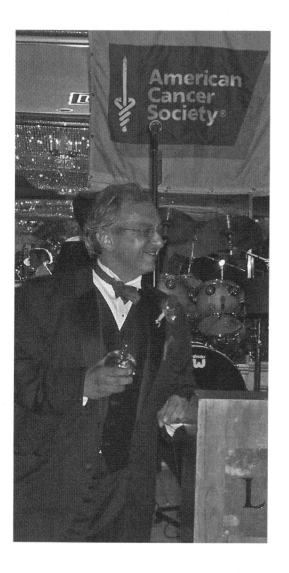

PRESS RELEASE

A Doctor is Honored. So What?!

When The American Cancer Society honors a doctor of integrative medicine, it IS a big deal.

New York City, NY – The American Cancer Society's Fourth Annual Big Apple Basket Ball of May 11, 2007, paid tribute to four individuals — but, one person stood out.

Bill Akpinar, MD, DDS, DrAc, PhD (Pain Management and Oriental Medicine), known as Dr. Bill, has more Eastern and Western credentials that could be listed here, but why boggle the mind? This man lives to heal, and does so from the understanding that individuals are mind, body, and spirit and that healing of any one, must address all three.

A testament to his passion and caring about his fellow man was shared by Don Hazelton who introduced Dr. Bill prior to receiving his award. Living just a few houses apart, Hazelton called Dr. Bill at 3a.m. when his son was a toddler and in medical distress. When Dr. Bill answered the phone and was told there was a problem, Hazelton waited to hear what the doctor advised. All he heard was silence. He said, "Bill? Bill?" - but heard nothing in reply. His wife said, "Forget Bill. Call 911!" Before Hazelton could hang up the phone, he heard someone pounding on his door. He opened it and there was Bill Akpinar, in his pajamas. He hadn't bothered to hang up his phone, just ran to his friend's house and successfully treated the little boy. As good as this story is, it's only one of thousands upon thousands about an individual committed to his purpose.

Dr. Bill spoke to the hundreds of attendees and summarized what actually triggers cancer or other diseases to develop, as well as the practical ways individuals can prevent or address any imbalance in the body, if one takes place. Though the other three individuals deserved to be honored for their contributions, Dr. Bill was the sole recipient of a standing ovation.

He continues to treat patients and train doctors in various protocols, but Dr. Bill has expanded his purpose as an educator through his highly-informative, yet reader-friendly books that comprise Dr. Bill's Health and Wellness Series.

For more information about his books or to arrange an interview or speaking engagement, please contact Dr. Bill Akpinar at 718.428.2780 or drakpinar@aol.com.